Clinical Cases in Dysfluency

Clinical Cases in Dysfluency is an imperative work that introduces dysfluency in clinical and cultural contexts while encouraging reflection on clinical decision-making involving the assessment and management of clients. With inputs from eminent clinical researchers across the world, this text brings together diverse voices and expertise to provide readers with innovative ideas for their own practice.

The book assists in refining clinical problem solving and valuing exchanges between clients and clinicians. Featuring real-life case studies covering stuttering and cluttering in children and adults, it showcases the importance of evidence-based practice and practitioner reflection, demonstrating a range of approaches to address problems experienced with dysfluency, and their management. The authors go on to discuss issues of stereotyping, resilience, and therapeutic commonalities in general, and in multicultural contexts, whilst also introducing the discipline of *Dysfluency Studies*, where stuttering is considered positively in its complexity and not as a disorder. These concepts are effectively further illustrated through accompanying online resources including videos, and weblinks.

This is an indispensable resource for students and clinicians in the domains of Fluency, Speech and Language Pathology and Communication Disorders, and will be valuable reading to anyone interested in communication disorders, dysfluencies, and application of theory to practice in these disciplines.

Kurt Eggers is a professor at Ghent University, Thomas More Antwerp, and Turku University. He is ECSF chair, IFA president, EFS secretary and associate editor for Journal of Fluency Disorders. He has worked clinically for many years and his research focuses on the role of temperament and executive functioning in stuttering and speech dysfluencies in different populations.

Margaret M. Leahy has been a clinical researcher and associate professor at Trinity College Dublin, Ireland. She has written extensively on dysfluency and education. She has also served as journal editor and on journal editorial committees for many years. She actively contributes to the European Clinical Specialization in Fluency disorders (ECSF).

Clinical Cases in Speech and Language Disorders

Clinical Cases in Speech and Language Disorders is a new series of short books that each focuses on a specific speech and language disorder, providing an in-depth look at real or imagined scenarios, and discussing relevant assessment and intervention plans using theory, research findings, and clinical reasoning. The overall aim of these books is to provide much-needed resources using real-life clinical cases to help clinicians and students reflect on clinical decision making involving the assessment and management of patients presenting with various speech and language disorders (SLD).

Titles in the series:

Clinical Cases in Dysarthria
Edited by Margaret Walshe and Nick Miller

Clinical Cases in Dysphagia
Edited by Margaret Walshe and Maggie-Lee Huckabee

Clinical Cases in Dysfluency
Edited by Kurt Eggers and Margaret M. Leahy

For more information about this series, please visit: https://www.routledge.com/Clinical-Cases-in-Speech-and-Language-Disorders/book-series/CCSLD

Clinical Cases in Dysfluency

Edited by Kurt Eggers and
Margaret M. Leahy

Routledge
Taylor & Francis Group

LONDON AND NEW YORK

Cover image: Getty

First published 2023
by Routledge
4 Park Square, Milton Park, Abingdon, Oxon OX14 4RN

and by Routledge
605 Third Avenue, New York, NY 10158

Routledge is an imprint of the Taylor & Francis Group, an informa business

British Library Cataloguing-in-Publication Data
A catalogue record for this book is available from the British Library

Library of Congress Cataloguing-in-Publication Data
A catalog record has been requested for this book

ISBN: 978-1-032-01537-8 (hbk)
ISBN: 978-1-032-01538-5 (pbk)
ISBN: 978-1-003-17901-6 (ebk)

DOI: 10.4324/9781003179016

Typeset in Bembo
by MPS Limited, Dehradun

Contents

Preface

As Series Editor of *Clinical Cases in Speech and Language Disorders*, I am delighted to introduce *Clinical Cases in Dysfluency* edited by professors Kurt Eggers and Margaret Leahy, both leading academic researchers in dysfluency. This book, aimed at a global audience of early career speech-language therapists/pathologists or clinicians new to dysfluency, promises to be a valuable resource for clinical teaching and problem-based learning.

As in the other texts in the *Clinical Cases in Speech and Language Disorders* series, the terms 'case report', 'case presentation', 'case study', are used prudently in this book. Unlike case studies, which tend to have an element of planning and control, case reports are unplanned. They are narrative based, used to describe events as they occurred in order to illustrate a specific point. Case reports often provide first line evidence for new interventions, novel approaches to management, or function as 'alarms', signalling that an issue may exist with an already established treatment. Despite the fact that case reports are considered of minor importance in the field of evidence-based practice, sitting at the bottom of the 'Evidence Pyramid', nonetheless, they are immensely important in helping us learn about the various facets of clinical practice. Case reports reflect real life clients, expose clinical conundrums, and give us valuable insight into clinical decision making. Each case report within this text serves to illustrate or expand on a specific clinical message or support a core argument.

This book brings together a wealth of information from international clinicians and researchers in dysfluency. The text presents case reports, spanning dysfluency in preschool children and adults to cluttering and acquired fluency disorders. As well as case reports, there are chapters on the processes of therapeutic change, commonalities in successful therapy, multicultural commonalities, and an introduction to 'Dysfluency Studies', where stuttering is considered positively in its complexity. I remain indebted to the editors and the authors of individual chapters for this highly valued contribution to the *Clinical Cases in Speech and Language Disorders* series.

Margaret Walshe
February 2022

Contributors

Charley Adams is a Speech-Language Pathologist who earned his PhD from the University of South Carolina, where he conducts clinical and classroom teaching on fluency disorders. He serves on the board of the National Stuttering Association, and received their Speech Pathologist of the Year award in 2014. Charley is the past chair of the International Cluttering Association.

Ali Berquez is Clinical Lead for Children at the Michael Palin Centre and a Registered European Fluency Specialist. As a qualified practitioner in CBT and SFBT, Ali integrates these methods clinically with clients who stutter and their parents. She contributes to the Centre's clinical work, teaching, writing and research. Recent publications have focused on expectations from therapy and desensitisation with parents.

Michael Blomgren is a professor and chair of the Department of Communication Sciences & Disorders at the University of Utah. He completed his B.Sc. in Psychology (University of Victoria), his M.S. in Speech Pathology (University of Hawaii), and his PhD in Communication Science (University of Connecticut). Dr. Blomgren's research interests are broadly focused in two areas: evaluating aspects of speech motor control in stuttering and nonstuttering speakers; evaluating treatment outcomes of stuttering treatment.

Courtney Byrd is a professor, and Founding/Executive Director of the Arthur M. Blank Center for Stuttering Education and Research, which has three core branches dedicated to research, training, and clinical practice: Michael and Tami Lang Stuttering Institute, Dealey Family Foundation Stuttering Clinic, and Dr. Jennifer and Emanuel Bodner Developmental Stuttering Lab. She developed and manualized Camp Dream. Speak. Live.

Sarah Caughter is a Highly Specialist Speech and Language Therapist at the MPC and a Registered European Fluency Specialist. She has an MSc in CBT with children and young people and is a 'Reaching In Reaching Out' trainer, supporting professionals in building resilience in children.

She contributes to the clinical, teaching and research programmes at the MPC and has published peer-reviewed journal articles on resilience in children who stutter.

Susanne Cook is a Speech-Language Pathologist who earned her PhD from University College London, with a special interest in fluency disorders. A certified stuttering therapist (ivs), she established and ran for ten years a children's intensive stuttering therapy program. Susanne co-authored the German evidence-based medical guidelines for fluency disorders, and currently serves as the chair of the International Cluttering Association.

Francesca Del Gado is an Italian Speech-Language Pathologist and a registered European Fluency Specialist. She is a lecturer in fluency disorders at Sapienza University of Rome. She works with CRC staff in development of the MIDA-SP approach: the Multidimensional, Integrated, Differentiated, Art-mediated Stuttering Program and Play! Program for early intervention with children who stutter.

Kurt Eggers is a professor at Ghent University, Thomas More Antwerp and Turku University. He is ECSF chair, IFA president, EFS secretary and associate editor for Journal of Fluency Disorders. Kurt has worked clinically for many years and his research focuses on the role of temperament and executive functioning in stuttering and speech dysfluencies in different populations.

Elaine Kelman is Consultant Speech-Language Therapist and Head of the Michael Palin Centre and a Registered European Fluency Specialist (EFS). She contributes to the Centre's development of stuttering therapy programmes, its training and research programme. Elaine is chair of the EFS Board, ASHA affiliate, Specialist Adviser to the RCSLT and is Secretary of the Executive Board of the International Fluency Association.

Margaret M. Leahy has been a clinical researcher and associate professor at Trinity College Dublin, Ireland. She has written extensively on dysfluency and clinical education, and has served as journal editor and on journal editorial committees for many years. She actively contributes to the European Clinical Specialization in Fluency disorders (ECSF).

Sharon Millard, Phd, is Research Lead and a Clinical Specialist at the Michael Palin Centre in London and lecturer at City University of London. Her research is clinically driven and largely focused on treatment efficacy and outcome measurement. She is currently Chief Investigator for an NIHR funded feasibility trial to investigate Palin Stammering Therapy for School aged Children.

Mary O'Dwyer, Phd, is a Specialist Speech-Language Therapist with a special interest in the stories told by people who stutter. She includes narrative practice as a main component in her work with people who stutter. She has researched and published on the topic and teaches other therapists and students about this approach.

R. Sertan Özdemir, Phd, is a Turkish Speech-Language Therapist, working as an assistant professor at Istanbul Medipol University (Turkey), SLT Department. He mainly lectures on fluency disorders and supervises graduate theses. He is an ECSF graduate (2014) and his clinical expertise is on fluency disorders.

Fiona Ryan, Phd, is a Specialist Speech-Language Therapist working with children, adolescents and adults who stutter. A graduate of the European Clinical Specialist Programme in Fluency disorders, research interests include outcomes from Narrative Therapy for people who stutter. She lectures on disorders of Fluency in TCD and UCC.

Selma Saad Merouwe is a Slovak-Lebanese Speech-Language Pathologist and a registered European Fluency Specialist. She is a lecturer in fluency disorders, studies coordinator, and thesis supervisor at Saint-Joseph University of Beirut. She is a PhD candidate at Turku University (Finland) and Saint-Joseph University (Lebanon). In her clinical practice and research, she focuses on fluency disorders and bilingualism.

Trudy Stewart, Phd, is a retired consultant Speech and Language Therapist who worked with children and adults who stammer for 40 years. Her last role was clinical lead of the Stammering Support Centre in Leeds. She taught specialist courses for clinicians internationally, including on ECSF courses. She has carried out clinical research and presented her work at international conferences. She has written several texts on stammering and recently co-wrote and directed a play about stammering called 'Unspoken'.

Maria Stuart is assistant professor, School of English, Drama and Film at University College Dublin, where her teaching and research are in American literature, crime fiction, and medical humanities. She is co-editor of a special issue of Journal of Interdisciplinary Voice Studies on dysfluency 5:2 (2021), and Principal Investigator for Wellcome-funded project 'Metaphoric Stammers and Embodied Speakers': Connecting Clinical, Cultural and Creative Practice in Dysfluent Speech.

John A. Tetnowski is the Jeanette Sias endowed chair in Communication Sciences and Disorders at Oklahoma State University. He has over 25 years of clinical experience and is a board-certified fluency specialist. He has published over 80 manuscripts in fluency disorders and research methods and is an ASHA Fellow. He is the 2021-2024 editor of Perspectives in Fluency Disorders.

Catherine Theys is a senior lecturer in the School of Psychology, Speech and Hearing at the University of Canterbury (New Zealand), where she directs the Master in Speech and Language Pathology programme. Her research focuses on the behavioural and neural characteristics of stuttering and acquired neurogenic communication disorders, with a specific interest in the diagnosis and treatment of acquired stuttering.

Sabine Van Eerdenbrugh works at Thomas More University of Applied Sciences (Antwerp, Belgium). She developed the Internet-based Lidcombe Program Training for her PhD at the Australian Stuttering Research Centre. Sabine specialises in stuttering but has treated a variety of disorders. She is a member of the Lidcombe Program Trainers Consortium and of EBPracticeNet at the Centre of Evidence-Based Medicine (Leuven, Belgium).

Veerle Waelkens is a fluency specialist (EFS) with extensive experience with fluency in a multi-disciplinary setting and private practice. She lectures in fluency and Speech at Artevelde University of Applied Sciences in Ghent (Belgium), and is an ECSF lecturer and coach for ECSF (European Clinical Specialization in Fluency disorders). She has authored books on Fluency and Childhood Apraxia of Speech. www.st-st-stotteren.be

Katarzyna Węsierska is an assistant professor at the University of Silesia (Poland) and a Speech-Language Therapist at the Logopedic Centre in Katowice. She is a registered European fluency specialist and an ECSF coach. Her research and clinical practice focus primarily on fluency disorders. Every two years, she co-organizes in Poland the International Conference of Logopedics: Fluency Disorders: Theory and Practice.

J. Scott Yaruss, is a professor of Communicative Sciences and Disorders at Michigan State University. He has published more than 100 peer-reviewed manuscripts and more than 300 other papers on stuttering, including the Overall Assessment of the Speaker's Experience of Stuttering (OASES) and several clinical guides (Stuttering Therapy Resources).

Abbreviations

ACT	Acceptance and Commitment Therapy
ASHA	American Speech, Language, and Hearing Association
CBT	Cognitive Behavioural Therapy
CampDSL	Camp Dream. Speak. Live
CELF	Clinical Evaluation of Language Fundamentals
CFT	Compassion Focused Therapy
CSI	Concealable Stigmatised Identity
DCM	Demands and Capacities Model
ECSF	European Clinical Specialization Fluency Disorders
EFS	European Fluency Specialists
FTS...FTS	Free To Stutter...Free To Speak
ICA	International Cluttering Association
LP	Lidcombe Program
MAR	Mean Articulation Rate
MSES	Metaphoric Stammers and Embodied Speakers
MiSP	Mindfulness in Schools Project
NATs	Negative Automatic Thoughts
NP	Narrative Practice
OASES	Overall Assessment of the Speaker's Experience of Stuttering
OD	Other Dysfluencies
PCI	Predictive Cluttering Inventory
Palin PCI	Palin Parent-Child Interaction
POSHA-S	Public Opinion Survey of Human Attributes—Stuttering
POSHA-Cl	Public Opinion Survey of Human Attributes—Cluttering
SLP	Speech Language Pathologist
SLT	Speech Language Therapy
SPA	Screening Phonological Accuracy
SFBT	Solution Focused Brief Therapy

SSI-4	Stuttering Severity Instrument-4
SLD	Stuttering-Like Dysfluencies
TPA-CC	Three-Pronged Approach to the Conceptualization of Cluttering
UUISC	University of Utah Intensive Stuttering Clinic
4S-scale	Self-Stigma of Stuttering Scale

1 Fluency, Disorders of Fluency, and Dysfluency

Margaret M. Leahy and Kurt Eggers

Fluency and Dysfluency

This book features clinical case reports regarding people who experience problems associated with the dysfluency characteristics of stuttering and cluttering. For speech and language clinicians[1] (hereafter: clinicians), the general classification of *Speech Disorders* incorporates fluency, articulation and voice disorders of different aetiologies. Stuttering and cluttering are classified as fluency disorders (e.g., Damico et al., 2021). A separate category of *Language Disorders* is closely associated, as speech is a form of language use; however, disorders of speech do *not* represent disorders of language, although they often co-occur (e.g., see Chapter 12).

For current purposes, the terms fluency and dysfluency as used in this book refer to aspects of continuity or flow of speech-in-interaction, in a person's first language. We regard fluency/dysfluency as a continuum, where both occur naturally in speech utterances. The term fluency (derives from Latin 'fluencia', 'fluere', to flow) designates smoothness, ease, connectedness, naturalness, regularity and rhythm (e.g., Starkweather, 1987). Whereas dysfluency represents occasional, variable, (often involuntary) breaks or interruptions in transitions or connectedness at any or all levels of phoneme, syllable, word and phrase utterances. Influences on the quality and quantity of the fluency/dysfluency continuum include speech rate, intonation, hesitations, interjections, and repetitions, all of which function in our communication repertoire as integral to how we develop our capacities in communicating, including speech production (e.g., Shapiro, 2011; Ward, 2006). This process begins rapidly and systematically during the initial years of life and continues well beyond this period, as it is influenced directly by elements that include biological, linguistic, and sociological factors, as well as by opportunities for interaction, and by cognitive and emotional processing. Walsh et al. (2017) capture its complexity succinctly: "Although seemingly effortless, fluent speech production is a remarkably complex process, requiring the functional synergy of multiple neural networks to accomplish language formulation, articulatory planning, motor execution, and auditory and somatosensory integration" (p. 1).

DOI: 10.4324/9781003179016-1

For the purposes of clinical work with individuals who experience problems associated with stuttering and cluttering, further defining elements are important. A hallmark of (observable) dysfluency is its variability, that can range from complete fluency (or absence of dysfluencies) to interrupted flow with each syllable spoken. The patterns of variability can be systematic for each person, so that dysfluency can be predicted, but this too is variable. Tichenor and Yaruss (2021) report that variability is among the most frustrating aspects of stuttering, and that it is experienced across behaviours, emotional and cognitive reactions. They consider that variability is a 'burdensome aspect of the experience of stuttering', and suggest that it is given better attention in assessment, therapy, and research. Gerlach et al. (2021) add to this that because of this variability, the 'stuttering identity' of people who stutter can be unnoticed by listeners and they can 'pass' as fluent speakers (Constantino et al., 2017).

Disorders of Fluency

Stuttering

A fluency disorder is defined by the American Speech, Language, and Hearing Association as "an interruption in the flow of speaking characterised by atypical rate, rhythm, and dysfluencies (e.g., repetitions of sounds, syllables, words, and phrases; sound prolongations; and blocks), which may also be accompanied by excessive tension, speaking avoidance, struggle behaviors, and secondary mannerisms (ASHA, 2022). Tichenor and Yaruss (2018) state that stuttering involves more than (dysfluency) behaviours identifiable by listeners: "definitions of stuttering based merely on the more superficial characteristics of dysfluencies may lead to evaluation protocols that are too narrow" (p. 1190). The same authors have recently suggested that the term 'fluency' is not fully inclusive, but that it is limiting and misleading, so that we should stop referring to stuttering as a fluency disorder and simply refer to it as stuttering (Tichenor et al., 2022).

Stuttering[2], the most common fluency disorder, is also designated as childhood onset fluency disorder (Diagnostic and Statistical Manual of Mental Disorders, 5th Ed.; American Psychiatric Association, 2013). Dysfluency characteristics of stuttering include involuntary sound or word repetitions, prolongations, and breaks between phonemes at syllable and at word levels, often uttered with associated effort or tension. This condition is typically accompanied by anxiety about speaking and can place limitations on how comfortable a child feels participating in social or academic environments. Because of these noticeable interruption phenomena in comparison with more fluent connected speech, and because it may be difficult to control, stuttering is generally recognisable as 'different', and has been recorded historically since at least c.2000BC in the early Egyptian hieroglyphics (Faulkner, 1976; in Shapiro, 2011; 2018). Its cause and treatment have been the subject of speculation and experimentation since early recorded medical history, with e.g., Hippocrates (450-357 BC) and Galen (131–201AD) among physicians contributing to discussions.

The typical age of stuttering onset is 2–3 years, and although c. 8% of preschool children start to stutter at a certain point in time (Yairi & Ambrose, 2013), up to 80% of children will recover (Yairi & Seery, 2015). The 20–25% who persist in stuttering "will struggle with a communication disorder that is resistant to treatment throughout their lives" (Walsh et al., 2017).

Factors contributing to causes of childhood stuttering are now known to include genetic and epigenetic factors, as well as factors related to linguistic functioning, childhood emotional (Eggers & Jones, 2022; Jones et al., 2022) and temperamental factors (Eggers et al., 2021), and developing sensorimotor processes (Smith & Weber, 2017). Smith and Weber conclude: "Although stuttering ultimately reflects impairment in speech sensorimotor processes, its course over the life span is strongly conditioned by linguistic and emotional factors" (p.3).

In addition to stuttering of childhood origin, the phenomena of adult-onset stuttering of idiopathic origin (Leahy & Stewart, 1997), pharmacogenic stuttering (Brady, 1998) and acquired stuttering of neurological origin (Theys & De Nil, 2022) have been documented (see Chapter 12).

Cluttering

Although the study of cluttering, once labelled as the 'orphan of speech-language pathology' (Daly, 1993), dates back almost 300 years, it is not as clearly defined or as well-known as stuttering (Duchan & Felsenfeld, 2021), possibly due to its considerably lower prevalence rates (Sommer et al., 2021). The dysfluency characteristics of cluttering include excessive typical dysfluencies (hesitations, interjections, repetitions), irregularity in speech rate, rhythm, stress or pausing, and frequent deletion or collapsing of syllables (see Chapter 10). In addition, stuttering features can appear with cluttering simultaneously. Cluttered speech is often described as 'too fast', 'unintelligible', or both, and it may occur inconsistently in a person's speech. Some have referred to it as a 'central language imbalance' (Weiss, 1964) or a syndrome (St. Louis et al., 2003) and the specific characteristics required for diagnoses (Daly & Cantrell, 2006; Van Zaalen et al., 2009; Ward, 2006) have been the topic of debate. The *lowest common denominator definition*, a definition that is currently broadly used, defines cluttering as a fluency disorder wherein segments of the speaker's conversation are perceived as too fast overall, too irregular, or both; in combination with excessive normal dysfluencies, collapsing or deletion of syllables, and/or abnormal pauses, syllable stress, or speech rhythm (St. Louis & Schulte, 2011).

Stereotype and Stigma

Stereotypes are over-generalised attitudes or exaggerated beliefs regarding groups of people, that are thought to assist in simplifying complex information about them. When we engage in stereotyping groups of people, we assign a range of characteristics and abilities (often negative) to the group, assuming that all members of the group share them. The stutterer stereotype is that people who stutter are nervous, untrustworthy, shy, insecure, introverted and self-conscious (e.g., Craig et al., 2003), as well as being less intelligent than people who do not stutter (e.g., Silverman & Paynter, 1990).

Studies regarding the stutterer stereotype show its pervasiveness in societies worldwide: St. Louis (2011; 2015) developed the Public Opinion Survey of Human Attributes—Stuttering (POSHA-S) and the Public Opinion Survey of Human Attributes—Cluttering (St. Louis et al., 2014) to measure public attitudes toward stuttering and cluttering. Its data represents opinions from individuals in five continents worldwide, demonstrating that the stereotype is more similar than different in diverse communities. Attitudes toward cluttering are similar to—but somewhat less positive than—attitudes toward stuttering (St. Louis et al., 2014). Differences in attitudes are influenced by factors that include e.g., education, socio-economic status, and contact with people who stutter and clutter.

Social effects of the stereotype include the possibility of bullying and unfair employment discrimination, as well as elements of social rejection, and in some instances, attracting pity from people (e.g., Boyle & Blood, 2015). Elevated levels of stutterers' anxiety can also be a factor related to anticipated negative listener reactions (e.g., Iverach & Rapee, 2014).

Stutterer Stigma

The stigma of stuttering is associated with the stereotype in that stigma represents a sign or stain that marks persons who stutter, effectively reducing their social power as stigma casts upon them a 'spoiled identity' that is 'deeply discrediting' (Goffman, 1963). This devalued identity not only reduces the social standing of the stigmatised group members, but can affect quality of life, with restricted opportunities across wide-ranging aspects of community functioning, including e.g., employment (Gabel et al., 2004) and education, as PWS are perceived to be less competent or intelligent than their fluent counterparts (Silverman & Bongey, 1997; Silverman & Paynter, 1990). St. Louis (2020) reports from a comparative POSHA study that stuttering is considered "…as less stigmatising than mental illness but more stigmatising than obesity." An important finding from this study is that a person's knowledge of and experience with stigmatised conditions can inform both clinical work and public awareness campaigns that deal with stigma.

Self-stigma refers to the persons' internalisation of the stereotypes and discrimination that society holds (Corrigan et al., 2009), so that they come to believe these negative attitudes and then react emotionally to these beliefs, e.g., with reduced self-esteem and self-efficacy. Applying this stigma model to stuttering, Boyle (2013a) developed of The Self-Stigma of Stuttering Scale (4 S; revised version, Boyle, 2015). In studies regarding its impact,

Boyle (2013b; Boyle & Blood, 2015) indicates that self-stigma can have detrimental effects on a person's psychological well-being, affecting wide-ranging areas of quality of life. Additionally, it can affect a person's stress levels, physical health, and health care satisfaction (Boyle & Fearon, 2018).

Concealable Stigma Identity

The variability of stuttering, and its relative unpredictability can lead people who stutter to be uncertain whether listeners can identify them as stutterers, with its stigma. This means that a stutterer's identity can be imperceptible and concealed at times. Gerlach et al. (2021) consider the cognitive burden of this *concealable stigmatised identity* (CSI) as an additional social disadvantage of stuttering, potentially influencing clients' psychological health. Among their findings is that the burden of CSI adversely impacts the quality of life of the people who stutter. Self-disclosure, a documented strategy to decrease the vulnerability to stereotype threat, has also been suggested as a clinical tool for people who stutter (Byrd et al., 2017; Croft & Byrd, 2021; see also Chapter 5).

Dysfluency Studies

Dysfluency Studies is an emerging C21 concept that uses the term *dysfluency* referring principally to stuttering dysfluency, and challenging the clinical interpretation of stuttering as a fluency disorder, or indeed as disorder of any kind. The generally negative literary and cultural narratives of stuttering dysfluency reflect stutterer stigma stereotypical attitudes and as noted, too often have a disabling impact when the stutterer meets with elements of social bias or rejection. Stuart (see Chapter 9) rightly asserts that these narratives need to be rewritten in the light of creative practices, moving towards dysfluency narratives of triumph that can be multi-layered and ultimately generative.

Therapy and Self-help Support Groups

The need for therapy depends on the age of the client, the severity of the fluency disorder, the impact on one's daily life and it is inherently linked to self-stigma. Some even argue stuttering therapy would no longer be needed if cultural responses to stuttering (and cluttering) would change and they are no longer considered as 'disordered speech' (see Chapter 9). Moreover, the content of therapy does not only depend on evidence-based practice, but is often determined by culturally determined, country-specific motives (Blomgren et al., 2019; see Chapter 9). In younger children, it is important to consider the possibility of natural recovery (Yairi & Ambrose, 2005) and both direct and indirect approaches in therapy (see Chapters 3 & 4). For older clients, there is a range of 'stutter-more-fluently' and 'speak-more-fluently' approaches (see Chapters 6, 7, & 8), and most would agree that therapy a collaborative journey with shared understanding, joint clinical decision-making, and therapeutic alliance between client and clinician (Eggers, 2021).

Van Riper's (1973; 1982) major textbook on the treatment of stuttering supported the argument for therapeutic approaches that stretched beyond stuttered speech to include the person's social, emotional and cognitive re-actions to it (see Chapter 7). Since then, therapies have developed and changed to incorporate research on the complex nature of dysfluency, providing evidence for successful outcomes, as well as diverse approaches, as demonstrated by the different case reports in this book.

Self-help support groups instigated and run by people who stutter help provide local, national and international meeting opportunities, as well as promoting awareness of stuttering, along with education, advocacy and research (see Chapter 11). They are often used as an adjunct to therapy (see Chapter 11), and may be an alternative to therapy for some. It is important to note that leaders of the self-help movement are shown to have more positive attitudes towards stuttering than members of other groups (St. Louis, 2020). These organisations have many advantages in recognising the stutterer's social communication needs, and in helping members improve their confidence. Boyle (2013b) indicates that support groups limit internalisation of negative attitudes, and thus, the possibility of reducing self-stigma, promoting higher levels of psychological well-being for members.

Outline of Chapters

The chapters that follow comprise a series of clinical case reports in aspects of dysfluency, including developmental and acquired stuttering and cluttering, along with a non-clinical chapter that introduces readers to re-writing cultural narratives of dysfluency, challenging the tradition of classifying stuttering as a disorder. Along with case reports, there are chapters that consider the process of therapeutic change (Chapter 2); Commonalities in working in therapies with evidence for success (Chapter 3); Stuttering therapy approaches (Chapter 7), and Commonalities in multicultural contexts (Chapter 11).

In the introduction to the first book in this series, Walshe and Huckabee (2019; 2) favour the use of *case reports* above case studies, pointing out that they "… tend not to be planned or controlled, but are rather a description of events as they occurred, in order to make a specific point". As such, case reports are naturalistic, they convey a key message, and they can provide a means of expanding hypotheses to explain observed phenomena. We echo their statement regarding the status of case reports that "… although considered the lowest form of evidence, the humble case report in some respects is the origin of new thinking." (p1).

The main types of case reports in this book comprise (a) Collective cases: where a series of cases simultaneously provide support for a particular argument (Chapters 4, 5, 6, & 10); (b) Evaluative case: to demonstrate how well a particular approach works (Chapter 8); and (c) Explanatory case: to provide in-depth understanding on a specific issue (Chapters 11 & 12). *Supplementary online material* is provided on an e-Resource page (at Routledge.co.uk).

Notes

1 The terms speech and language therapist, speech-language pathologist, and logopedist are terms that are used worldwide interchangeably and, in this book, also the term clinician is used.
2 Stuttering and stammering are synonymous terms, used interchangeably.

References

American Psychiatric Association. (2013). *Diagnostic and statistical manual of mental disorders* (5th Ed.). Washington, DC: The Policy Press.

American Speech-Language-Hearing Association (n.d.). Fluency Disorders (Practice Portal). Retrieved Jan 15th 2022, from www.asha.org/practice-portal/clinical-topics/fluency-disorders/

Blomgren, M., Eggers, K., Packman, A., & Azios, M. (2019, August). *Stuttering treatment: Trending issues and global resources.* Lecture presented at the 31st World Congress of the International Association of Logopedics and Phoniatrics, Taipei, Taiwan.

Boyle, M. P. (2013a). Assessment of stigma associated with stuttering: Development and evaluation of the self-stigma of stuttering scale (4S). *Journal of Speech, Language, and Hearing Research.* 56, 1517–1529. 10.1044/1092-4388(2013/12-0280

Boyle, M. P. (2013b). Psychological characteristics and perceptions of stuttering of adults who stutter with and without support group experience. *Journal of Fluency Disorders.* 38 (4), 368–381. 10.1016/j.jfludis.2013.09.001

Boyle, M. P. (2015). Identifying correlates of self-stigma in adults who stutter: Further establishing the construct validity of the Self-Stigma of Stuttering Scale (4S). *Journal of Fluency Disorders.* 43, 17–27. 10.1016/j.jfludis.2014.12.002

Boyle, M. P. & Blood, G. W. (2015). Stigma and stuttering: Conceptualizations, applications, and coping. In K. O. St. Louis (Ed.), *Stuttering meets stereotype, stigma, and discrimination: An overview of attitude research* (pp. 43–70). Morgantown, WV: West Virginia University Press.

Boyle, M. P. & Fearon, A. N. (2018). Self-stigma and its associations with stress, physical health, and health care satisfaction in adults who stutter. *Journal of Fluency Disorders.* 56, 112–112. 10.1016/j.jfludis.2017.10.0

Brady, J. P. (1998). Drug-induced stuttering: A review of the literature. *Journal of Clinical Psychopharmacology.* 18 (1), 50–54. 10.1097/00004714-199802000-00008

Byrd, C. T., Croft, R., Gkalitsiou, Z., & Hampton, E. (2017). Clinical utility of self-disclosure for adults who stutter: Apologetic versus informative statements. *Journal of Fluency Disorders.* 54, 1–13. 10.1016/j.jfludis.2017.09.001

Constantino, C. D., Manning, W. H., & Nordstrom, S. N. (2017). Rethinking covert stuttering. *Journal of Fluency Disorders.* 53, 26–40. 10.1016/j.jfludis.2017.06.001

Corrigan, P. W., Larson, J. E., & Rüsch, N. (2009). Self-stigma and the "why try" effect: Impact on life goals and evidence-based practices. *World Psychiatry.* 8, 75–81. 10.1002/j.2051-5545.2009.tb00218.x

Craig, A., Tran, Y., & Magali, C. (2003). Stereotypes towards Stuttering for Those Who Have Never Had Direct Contact with People Who Stutter: A Randomized and Stratified Study. *Perceptual and Motor Skills.* 97(1), 235–245. 10.2466/PMS.97.5.235-245

Croft, R.L. & Byrd, C. T. (2021). Does the clinical utility of self-disclosure of stuttering transcend culturally and linguistically diverse populations? *International Journal of Speech and Language Pathology.* 23 (5), 548–558. 10.1080/17549507.2020.1861326

Daly, D. A. (1993). Cluttering: The Orphan of Speech-Language Pathology. *American Journal of Speech-Language Pathology.* 2, 6–8. 10.1044/1058-0360.0202.06

Daly, D. A. & Cantrell, R. P. (2006, July). *Cluttering characteristics identified as diagnostically significant by 60 fluency experts.* Paper presented at the International Fluency Congress Dublin, Ireland.

Damico, J. S., Müller, N., & Ball, M. J. (2021). *The Handbook of Language and Speech Disorders* (2nd Ed.). Chichester: Wiley-Blackwell.

Duchan, J. F. & Felsenfeld, S. (2021). Cluttering Framed: An Historical Overview. *Advances in Communication and Swallowing*, pre-press, 1–11. 10.3233/ACS-210029

Eggers, K. (2021). Stawanie się efektywnym logopedą specjalizującym się w zaburzeniach płynności mowy [Becoming an effective clinician specialized in fluency disorders]. In K. Wesierska & H. Sönsterud (Eds.) *Dialog bez barier – kompleksowa interwencja w jąkaniu. Wydanie polskie rozszerzone [Dialogue without barriers: Comprehensive stuttering management].* (pp. 65–83). Katowice: University of Silesia.

Eggers, K. & Jones, R. (2022). Temperament, emotions and stuttering. In D. Tomaiuoli (Eds.), *Proceedings of the 4th international conference on stuttering.* Trento: Erickson.

Eggers, K., Millard, S., & Kelman, E. (2021). Temperament and the impact of stuttering in adolescents. *Journal of Speech, Language, and Hearing Research.* 64, 417–432.

Faulkner, R. O. (1976). A concise dictionary of Middle Egyptian. Oxford: Griffith Institute. In Shapiro, D. A. , *Stuttering intervention: A collaborative journey to fluency freedom* (2nd Ed.) Austin, Texas: Pro-Ed.

Gabel, R. M., Blood, G. W., Tellis, G. M., & Althouse, M. T. (2004). Measuring role entrapment of people who stutter. *Journal of Fluency Disorders.* 29(1), 27–49. 10.1016/j.jfludis.2003.09.002

Gerlach, H., Chaudoir, S. R., & Zebrowski, P. M. (2021). Relationships between stigma-identity constructs and psychological health outcomes among adults who stutter. *Journal of Fluency Disorders.* 70, 105842. 10.1016/j.jfludis.2021.105842

Goffman, E. (1963). *Stigma: Notes on the management of spoiled identity.* Englewood Cliffs, NJ: Prentice-Hall.

Iverach, L. & Rapee, R. M. (2014). Social anxiety disorder and stuttering: Current status and future directions. *Journal of Fluency Disorders.* 40, 69–82. 10.1016/j.jfludis.2013.08.003

Jones, R., Eggers, K., & Zengin-Bolatkale, H. (July 2022). Temperamental and emotional processes. In P. Zebrowski, J. Anderson, and E. Conture (Eds.) *Stuttering: Characteristics, assessment, and treatment* (4th Ed.). Thieme Medical Publishers.

Leahy M.M., & Stewart T. (1997). Idiopathic Stuttering Onset in Adults. In Y. Lebrun (Ed.), *From the Brain to the Mouth. Neuropsychology and Cognition (Vol 12).* Dordrecht: Springer. 10.1007/978-94-011-5776-6_8

Silverman, F. H. & Bongey, T. A. (1997). Nurses' attitudes toward physicians who stutter. *Journal of Fluency Disorders.* 22, 61–62. 10.1016/S0094-730X(96)00056-3

Silverman, F. H. & Paynter, K. K. (1990). Impact of stuttering on perception of occupational competence. *Journal of Fluency Disorders.* 15, 87–91. 10.1016/0094-730X(90)90035-Q

Shapiro, D. A. (2011). *Stuttering Intervention: A Collaborative Journey to Fluency Freedom* (2nd Ed). Austin, Texas: Pro-Ed.

Smith, A. & Weber, C. (2017). How Stuttering Develops: The Multifactorial Dynamic Pathways Theory. *Journal of Speech, Language, and Hearing Research.* 60, 2483–2505. 10.1044/2017_JSLHR-S-16-0343. PMID: 28837728.

Sommer, M. Waltersbacher, A., Schlotmann, A., Schröder, H., & Strzelczyk, A. (2021). Prevalence and Therapy Rates for Stuttering, Cluttering, and Developmental Disorders of Speech and Language: Evaluation of German Health Insurance Data. *Frontiers in Human Neuroscience.* 15, 645292. 10.3389/fnhum.2021.645292

Starkweather, C. W. (1987). *Fluency and stuttering.* Englewood Cliffs, NJ: Prentice–Hall.

St. Louis, K. O. (2011). The Public Opinion Survey of Human Attributes-Stuttering (POSHA–S): Summary framework and empirical comparisons. *Journal of Fluency Disorders.* 36, 256–261. 10.1016/j.jfludis.2011.02.003

St. Louis, K. O. (2015). Epidemiology of public attitudes toward stuttering. In K. O. St. Louis (Ed.), *Stuttering meets stereotype, stigma, and discrimination: An overview of attitude research* (pp. 7–42). Morgantown, WV: West Virginia University Press.

St. Louis, K. O. (2020). Comparing and Predicting Public Attitudes Toward Stuttering, Obesity, and Mental Illness. *American Journal of Speech-Language Pathology.* 29(4), 2023–2038. https://pubs.asha.org/doi/full/10.1044/2020_AJSLP-20-00038

St. Louis, K. O., Raphael, L. J., Myers, F. L., & Bakker, K. (2003). Cluttering updated. *The ASHA Leader.* 8-21 (November), 4–5 & 20–23. 10.1044/leader.FTR1.08212003.4

St. Louis, K. O., & Schulte, K. (2011). Defining cluttering: The lowest common denominator. In D. Ward, & K. Scaler Scott (Eds.), *Cluttering: a handbook of research, intervention and education* (pp. 233–253). Hove: Psychology Press. 10.4324/9780203 833421-26

St. Louis, K. O., Sonsterud, H., Carlo, E. J., Heitmann, R. R., & Kvenseth, H. (2014). Public attitudes toward and identification of cluttering and stuttering in Norway and Puerto Rico. *Journal of Fluency Disorders.* 42, 21–34. 10.1016/j.jfludis.2014.05.005

Theys, C. & De Nil, L.F. (July 2022). Acquired stuttering: etiology, symptomatology, identification and treatment. In P. Zebrowski, J. Anderson, and E. Conture (Eds.), *Stuttering: Characteristics, assessment, and treatment* (4th Ed.). Thieme Medical Publishers.

Tichenor, S. E., Constantino, C., & Yaruss, J. S. (2022). A Point of View About Fluency. *Journal of Speech, Language, and Hearing Research,* ePub ahead of issue, 10.1044/2021_JSLHR-21-00342

Tichenor, S. E. & Yaruss, J. S. (2018). A Phenomenological analysis of the experience of stuttering. *American Journal of Speech and Language Pathology.* 27, 1180–1194. 10.1044/2018_AJSLP-ODC11-17-0192

Tichenor, S. E. & Yaruss, J. S. (2021). Variability of Stuttering: Behavior and Impact. *American Journal of Speech-Language Pathology.* 30(1), 75–88. 10.1044/2020_AJSLP-20-00112

Van Riper, C. (1973). *The treatment of stuttering.* New Jersey: Prentice-Hall.

Van Riper, C. (1982). *The nature of stuttering.* New Jersey: Prentice-Hall.

Van Zaalen, Y., Wijnen, F., & De Jonckere, P. (2009). Differential diagnostic characteristics between cluttering and stuttering - Part one. *Journal of Fluency Disorders.* 34, 137–154. 10.1016/j.jfludis.2009.07.001

Walsh, F., Tian, J. A., Tourville, M. A., Yücel, T. K. & Bostian, A. J. (2017). Hemodynamics of speech production: An fNIRS investigation of children who stutter. *Scientific Reports.* 7, 4034.

Walshe, M. & Huckabee, M. (2019). *Clinical Cases in Dysphagia*. New York: Routledge.

Ward, D. (2006). *Stuttering and cluttering: Frameworks for understanding and treatment*. Hove: Psychology Press.

Weiss, D. A. (1964). *Cluttering*. Englewood Cliffs, NJ: Prentice-Hall.

Yairi, E., & Ambrose, N. G. (2005). *Early Childhood Stuttering for Clinicians by Clinicians*. Pennsylvania State University: PRO-ED.

Yairi, E., & Ambrose, N. (2013). Epidemiology of stuttering: 21st century advances. *Journal of Fluency Disorders*. 38(2), 66–87. 10.1016/j.jfludis.2012.11.002

Yairi, E., & Seery, C. H. (2015). *Stuttering: Foundations and Clinical Applications*. (2nd ed.) Pearson.

Yaruss, J. S., Quesal, R. W. (2004). Stuttering and the International Classification of Functioning, Disability, and Health (ICF): An update. *Journal of Communication Disorders*. 37(1), 35–52. 10.1016/S0021-9924(03)00052-2

2 Therapeutic Change: Models and Processes

Trudy Stewart

Change

A key concept in definitions of change is the notion of difference i.e., to make or become new, and to engage in a refreshingly different experience. However, the definitions fail to reflect the complexity of the process. Change involves an interplay between cognition/thoughts, feelings/emotions and behaviours. A change in one of these areas will impact on the other two (Figure 2.1).

For example, I decide to join a choir (a behaviour change). As a result of attending, I feel better; more connected socially and more energised (an emotional change). I think joining a choir is time well spent (a change in my thinking). Feeling better, I continue to attend the choir (the change in emotions feeds back into the behaviour change) and because I now believe that choirs in general are a 'good thing', my behaviour change and feelings are continually validated.

In this example I made a choice about making a change. This raises a number of issues about the role the self plays in a change process:

First, does the individual play a part in bringing about the difference? There are some change processes which take place largely without a person playing an active role. For example, the aging process involves many changes to our bodies and minds but we can do little to halt these naturally occurring alterations. Then there are other types of change which in-dividuals choose to engage in; these can involve changes to behaviours (gym attendance, learning to paint), to thinking (travelling abroad or living within a different culture) and feelings (practicing self-compassion, anxiety control techniques).

Second, does the person have an awareness of change? There may be instances of change which happen without a person being aware of its oc-currence. For example, an individual is usually immediately aware of something different in his mouth; a chipped tooth or a sore spot on the gums. In contrast, weight gain or loss is often something that a person notices gradually over time.

Finally, does the person have a psychological response to change? The answer relates to the amount the individual has 'invested' in what has

DOI: 10.4324/9781003179016-2

COGNITIONS

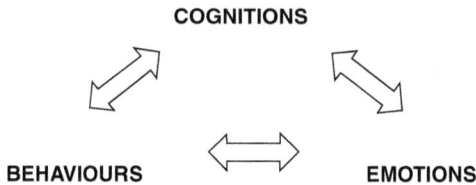

BEHAVIOURS   **EMOTIONS**

Figure 2.1 Interplay between cognitions, emotions and behaviours.

changed and/or how he feels or construes the change. If wearing the latest fashion item is important to a teenager, then being forced to don an unfashionable outfit for an adult function could be quite upsetting, especially if he/she is seen by their peers. However, for another young person for whom clothing is purely functional, this experience of change has little or no impact.

For some people the notion of change is something they will resist, preferring to keep the status quo. This, however, is an unnatural state, as change is happening constantly through developmental, cultural and social processes and in relationships.

Change and Stammering Therapy

Unquestionably therapy is about change; specifically, therapy formalises the change process. When an adult arrives for a therapy session wanting to address an issue with the help of a clinician, there is an unspoken contract that the therapy process will move him from his point of arrival to another place which will be different in some way. His previous and ongoing experience of change may be significant in relation to how he feels he is able to make and maintain change (see Craig, Franklin & Andrews, 1984) and how he engages in therapy. Positive past experiences of making change, which could include attending therapy previously, will result in positive anticipation of this therapy. If there are ongoing issues in his life which require change, such as relationship difficulties or major career shifts then this could affect his ability to engage in yet another change process.

The clinician may also be affected by her previous and ongoing experience of change and should be mindful of how her own construing could impact upon the therapy with clients. A clinician should also expect to be altered by her interaction with a client; she will learn a new narrative about stammering, experiment with some therapeutic and/or counselling techniques, learn what works and what is less successful for each person, reflect on her experiences and modify her practice as a result (see Stewart & Leahy, 2010; 2021).

While preparing to see an individual in order to facilitate an openness to change, a clinician might consider the following:

- Am I ready? What do I need to do to make sure I am fully present with this individual?
- Has the person chosen therapy himself, or been referred at the request of someone else (e.g., his employer, his partner, a friend)? How long has he been waiting for therapy and has anything happened in that time?
- Can I set aside any pre-emptions I have about persons of this age, gender, etc. and be open to this particular individual?
- Have I over-planned the session or left space to listen to what he has to say and together with him formulate a plan of how to move forward?

Stages of Change

An adult who stammers can be at different stages of change when coming to therapy. Judd, a young man who stammered since he was a boy, was referred by his doctor for therapy. He had a wide group of friends who supported him; they did his shopping, took him out, ordered for him in cafes. In short, they did almost everything for him and Judd had little need to communicate outside this circle of friends. Judd was aware of his stammer but had no motivation for change; indeed to do so may have jeopardised the convenient arrangements that were in place. This example illustrates the need for a clinician to ascertain at the beginning of a therapy where an individual might be in relation to the change process. It is wrong to assume that a person will be ready to embark upon significant modifications. As Judd showed, the desire for alterations may come from an external rather than internal source.

Secondly, there needs to be a match between the person's readiness to change and appropriate clinical intervention or self-help strategies. When a clinician understands where an individual is, she can help to move him through a particular stage with an intervention that matches where he is in his process.

Models of Change

Fishbein and Ajzen (1975) rejected general notions such as self-esteem or locus of control to explain why people behaved in certain ways. They suggested focusing on a particular behaviour and identifying what might predict and explain that specific behaviour. The reasoned action model (1975) states briefly that the principal determinant of a behaviour is the individual's intention to carry out that specific behaviour. The *model of reasoned action* was applied to the acquisition of fluent speech in a group of adults who stammered (Stewart, 1982). Results supported the relationships proposed by the model and showed a significant correlation between pre-therapy attitude and intention scores and fluency gains.

With links to Fishbein and Ajzen's work, the *transtheoretical or stages of change model* (Prochaska & DiClemente 1982; Prochaska, DiClemente & Norcross, 1992) tries to explain how an individual develops an intention to change.

This is done by delineating: "specific constellations of attitudes, intentions and behaviors that are relevant to an individual's status in the process of change" (p.5) (Prochaska & DiClemente 1992).

The model has been applied to a great many health related behaviours and also some applications to stammering, both in adults and children. Turnbull (2000) was the first clinician to describe the processes, levels and stages of change as described in Prochaska and DiClemente's work and apply these directly to work with adults with dysfluent speech. More recently Floyd et al. (2007) assessed the validity of the stages model and looked at the use of a modified version of the stages of change questionnaire with adults who stammered.

In trying to understand what the process of change or intention to change was, including a person's readiness to engage, Prochaska and DiClemente developed an assessment that revealed 6 stages of change (see Freeman & Dolan 2001 for an interesting expansion of the model). *(See online resource for a simple table summarising the stages, presentation, blocks to change and therapeutic strategies)*

Precontemplation

A person in this stage fails to acknowledge the need to think/feel or behave differently. This maybe because of lack of awareness of a problem, denial that a difficulty exists, feeling that he is unwilling or unable to carry out any modifications (This could be as a result of previous failures when attempts to change have been made). If an individual presents for therapy at this stage it is usually because some other person has an awareness of the problem, perhaps an employer or "significant other" in his life. Such a "coerced" individual would usually cease to attend after one or two sessions.

According to DiClemente (1991) an individual maybe stuck at this stage due to 4 possibilities: a) reluctance – frequently due to inertia or lack of knowledge; b) rebellion – there is some reason to maintain the problem and to keep the status quo; c) resignation – change is not seen as a possibility and there is an acceptance of living in a problem state; and d) rationalisation – the problem is not seen as the person's responsibility, rather it belongs to others. Understanding each of these reasons allows the clinician to present strategies as a counter response in her attempts to move the client on. The following interventions are suggested: a) empathy and appropriate feedback in response to reluctance; b) providing choices and the careful use of paradox in response to rebellion; c) instilling hope and exploring those issues that the client sees as barriers to change in response to resignation and d) Prochaska et al. (1992) suggest assessing feelings and encouraging thinking about the problem in relation to the self.

Turnbull (2000) notes the need for precontemplators to "own" the problem and paradoxically discusses 'no treatment' as an option to enable individuals to move forward: "Perhaps when we are presented with a precontemplator and feel attempts to move them on are likely to or have already failed, we should be more prepared to terminate therapy but to always leave the "therapy room door" open, so that clients know we are there to work with them when they are ready." (p17).

Contemplation

A person in this stage has moved to an acceptance that there is a problem to be solved. This may be due to a change in circumstances (e.g., a career move, a change in a relationship, marriage or birth of a child), but this must be accompanied by a change in intention if he is to progress further. The individual remains somewhat ambivalent about what to do to solve the situation and as Baldwin (1991) states: it is a "thinking not doing" stage. (p. 39). He remains fearful of the status quo and also future change. Consequently, it is an uncomfortable place to be but not one to be pushed or pulled out of, therapeutically speaking.

   Case example: Philip came for a therapy session having discovered he was to be a father for the first time. This news had created a number of anxieties for him: thoughts of having to read bedtime stories, parents' evenings at school, even a "father of the bride/groom" speech had been imagined. He described coping with his stammer primarily using avoidance but envisaged a time when this would fail him. He was anxious when he thought of the future but equally fearful of trying to change his current coping strategies.

   Intervention at this stage consisted of observation and identification of his stammer in day-to-day situations, discussion and guided reading around therapy options and perhaps most importantly, a meeting with another father. The father described to Philip how he talked about his stammer and how he coped with it with his young son, Isaac, as a way of empowering Isaac to manage some issues that he was facing in his young life.

   Useful therapy strategies are: a) motivational interviewing, which allows the person to understand his ambivalence and move to decision making (Miller & Rollnick, 1991); and b) self-evaluation techniques. These are specifically those which enable an individual to look at the implications of change, to weigh up the pros and cons of both staying the same and of change. Prochaska et al. (1992) also suggest a) increasing information about the self and the problem through observations, confrontations, interpretations and directed reading; and b) enabling the client to assess how he feels and thinks about himself with respect to the problem (i.e., consciousness raising).

Preparation

This is a stage during which behaviour intention develops; with both intention and attempts at behaviour change. It may be brief and it is important to recognise the readiness and capitalise upon it, otherwise the individual may move back to previous stages. Miller and Rollnick (1991) describe features of this stage:

- decreased questioning about change and less resistance to the problem,
- increased resolve and questions about change,
- more self-motivational statements and experimentation and
- some anticipation of life after the change has taken place.

It is often at this stage that a person who stammers will research interventions or go to the referral agent and ask for therapy. He may even attempt to make some changes to his speech e.g., changing his breathing or speaking rate.

Therapy strategies suggested by Prochaska and DiClemente (1992) include: a) enabling the client to assess how he feels and thinks about himself with respect to the problem (i.e., consciousness raising); and b) helping the individual to choose and commit to an act of change through decision making processes, making resolutions and commitment enhancing techniques.

Turnbull (2000) states that self-liberation is the key intervention at this stage. Thus, encouraging and helping an individual to believe he can make change is crucial. This can be done experientially by having the person identify some small change he can make; perhaps an observational task, such as noting the communication skills of a work colleague or friend. In a subsequent therapy session, the observations can be discussed in relation to how communication can be improved through a more holistic approach rather than focus on fluency.

Alternatively, the experiment could involve changing a routine activity, e.g., taking a different route to work, eating more slowly. Following this, a discussion may include how the change felt in the first instance and then over time, how the person remembered to make the change and what needed to happen for it to be maintained. The outcomes of such an experiment have direct implications for the next stage and the individual and clinician will note and reflect upon what has been learned.

Action

The action stage is one in which there is an awareness of cognitive, emotional and/or behaviour change. Examples could include changes from negative thoughts to more positive self-affirming thoughts, increased control over anxiety, and more openness about stammering and/or changes in the overall severity of stammering. Such changes may be observed by a clinician or an individual's 'significant other' or may only be noticed by the person himself.

The clinician's role in this stage is to present choices or alternatives from which the person can choose to experiment. For example, when experimenting with word avoidance Michael liked to have a number of options for different people and situations during the day:

a   specific person – saying what I want to say in conversations with my wife;
b   specific conversation – saying what I want to say when mentoring Pete, my colleague, at work (a daily conversation);
c   specific avoidance – noting specific words I avoid and working them back into sentences; and
d   openness – being open about avoidance, by saying 'I don't mean that. What I really meant to say was xxx'.

It is important that this experimentation is continued for as long as productive. Using a Personal Construct approach (Kelly, 1955, Hayhow & Levy, 1989; Fransella & Dalton, 1990; Stewart & Birdsall, 2001), a 'loose' approach to experimentation has been found to facilitate long term change (Stewart, 1996). Within the action stage the person may have peaks and troughs of motivation, as he is challenged or validated during this process. Fisher (2012) talked about the experience of specific emotional states along a 'personal transitional curve' (see online resources). In addition, this stage can be a precarious place for a client. There are those adults who stammer who embrace their experience and appear to be 'released' from the doubt that any change was impossible. Frequently there are those who move the therapy goal posts, realising that not only x is possible, but y and z may also be within reach. For others, the same experience of what is possible is anxiety producing and can send them running for the door. These individuals have found some aspects of stammering a safe haven which has sheltered them from certain situations/feelings/attainments. Now the option of moving from the safe haven raises fear and dread. These two alternatives, from many individual possibilities, show that a clinician needs to be alert to how the person is reacting to change and its options for their life.

As therapy strategies, Turnbull (200) states that self-liberation, counter conditioning, stimulus control and contingency management are all helpful processes for this stage. She specifies a number of stammering therapy options in relation to these areas. For example, counter conditioning – desensitisation, relaxation and assertiveness training would be relevant to 'toughen' an individual to adverse reactions, and negative thoughts or emotions. As for stimulus control, she suggests increased openness about stammering, and enlisting others to act as triggers or reminders to an adult who stammers to act in the way he intends. Contingency management involves building in rewards for when desired changes are made.

Turnbull also describes the clinician's role in this stage as gradually moving to a consultant as the individual takes increasing control over the changes he is making. The involvement of other important persons in the client's life and the support of a therapy group and/or self-help group can also facilitate change at this point.

Maintenance

Interestingly, Prochaska et al. (1992) accept that movement through the stages of change is not linear but more cyclical, with relapse being a natural part of the cycle. When relapse occurs, an individual can be prepared, will have learned from his journey through the change process and will tend to move through each stage again more quickly.

Maintenance can be an active stage in preparing for relapse in which a person is working on tried and tested strategies which keeps his change in place. The key therapy process here is the creation of an individual 'tool box' of strategies. However, the development of useful resources and ideas needs to be carried out from the outset of therapy and not left to the end stage. An adult or young person should be encouraged to collect and document his 'tools' as he progresses. This will enable him to write a summary at this maintenance stage, which can be shared with others and kept as a record of his work. (For more detailed description of *tool boxes and their development* and *a completed tool box* see Turnbull & Stewart, 2010).

A grid for the development of an individual tool box is included in the on-line resources.

Termination

This stable state is said to be characterised by a new self-image, no temptation to relapse, solid self-efficacy and healthier life style (Turnbull, 2000). It is useful to consider termination in the context of when an individual is moving away from therapy. A person often knows when he is ready and will convey this to the therapist in a number of ways. He may describe how he has em-barked on a new project, joined a social group or some other activity which is going to take up time and energy. For example, Gareth said he could no longer attend the therapy group as he had joined a sailing club and Zoe had taken the opportunity to extend her working hours.

As discussed in Stewart and Richardson (2004), adults who stammer frequently prefer ongoing and/or periodic support. This is often difficult to deliver in the context of time-limited service delivery. However, the place for an email, telephone or facetime review session can often pre-empt the need for longer term therapy and can actively prevent relapse. In addition, Linklater (2021) discusses a number of resources that a client could be signposted to by a clinician including websites, newsletters, national and international conferences on stammering, International Stuttering Awareness Day on line conference.

Conclusion

In this chapter models concerned in the process of change are discussed. Their relevance to the work carried out by an adult or young person who stammers and clinician in therapy should not be underestimated. The stages of change model can help a clinician choose an appropriate strategy to enable an individual to move forward and into active change. This improves outcomes and efficacy of therapy. In particular, this model details the cyclical nature of change and acknowledges an individual's need to move through stages perhaps numerous times at differing rates. With this understanding, relapse is seen as an important learning process and not a failure for either the person who stammers or the clinician. Such a positive approach to change can only benefit the work carried out in the clinic room and beyond.

References

Baldwin, S. (1991). Helping the unsure. In R. Davidson, S. Rollnick & I. McEwan (eds.), *Counselling Problem Drinkers.* London: Routledge.

Craig, A. R., Franklin, J. A., & Andrews, G. (1984). A scale to measure locus of control behaviour. *British Journal of Medical Psychology.* 57 (2), 173–180. 10.1111/j.2044-8341.1984.tb01597.x

DiClemente, C. C. (1991). Motivational interviewing and the stages of change. In W. R. Miller and S. Rollnick (eds.), *Motivational Interviewing.* New York: Guilford Press.

Fishbein, M. & Ajzen, I. (1975). *Belief, Attitude, Intention & Behavior.* Reading, M.A.: Addison-Wesley.

Fisher, J. (2012). The process of transition. www.businessballs.com

Floyd, J., Zebrowski. & Flamme, G. (2007). Stages of change and stuttering: A preliminary view. *Journal of Fluency Disorders.* 32, 95–120. 10.1016/j.jfludis.2007.03.001

Fransella, F. & Dalton, P. (1990). *Personal Construct Psychology in Action.* London: Sage.

Freeman, A. & Dolan, M. (2001). Revisiting Prochaska and DiClemente's stages of change theory: An expansion and specification to aid in treatment planning and outcome evaluation. *Cognitive and Behavioral Practice.* 8, 224–234. 10.1016/S1077-7229(01)80057-2

Hayhow, R. & Levy, C. (1989). *Working with Stuttering.* Bicester, Oxon: Winslow Press.

Kelly, G. A. (1955). *The Psychology of Personal Constructs: Vol 1 & 2.* New York: WW Norton. Co.

Linklater, J. (2021). Service Delivery. In T. Stewart. (ed.), *Stammering Resources for Adults & Teenagers: Integrating new evidence into clinical practice.* London: Routledge.

Miller, W. R. & Rollnick, S. (1991). *Motivational Interviewing.* New York: Guilford Press.

Prochaska, J. O. & DiClemente, C. C. (1982). Transtheoretical therapy: Toward a more integrative model of change. *Psychotherapy Theory Research and Practice.* 20, 161–173. https://doi.org/10.1037/h0088437

Prochaska, J. O. & DiClemente, C. C. (1992). Stages of change in the modification of problem behaviors. In M. Herson, R.M. Eisler & P. M. Miller (eds.), *Progress in Behavior Modification* volume 28. Illinois: Sycamore

Prochaska, J. O., DiClemente, C. C., & Norcross, J. C. (1992). In search of how people change: Applications to addictive behaviors. *American Psychologist.* 47, 1102–1114. 10.1037//0003-066x.47.9.1102

Stewart, T. (1982). The relationship of attitudes and intentions to behave to the acquisition of fluent speech behaviour by stammerers. *British Journal of Disorders of Communication.* 17, 3–13. 10.3109/13682828209012215

Stewart, T. (1996). Good maintainers and poor maintainers: a personal construct approach to an old problem. *Journal of Fluency Disorders*, 11, 22–48. 10.1016/0094-730x(95)00043-7

Stewart, T. & Birdsall, M. (2001). A review of the contribution of personal construct psychology to stammering therapy. *Journal of Constructivist Psychology*. 14, (3), 215–225. 10.1080/10720530126270

Stewart, T. & Leahy, M. M. (2021). The art and practice of being a clinician working with individuals who stammer. In T. Stewart (ed.), *Stammering Resources for Adults and Teenagers*. London: Routledge.

Stewart, T. & Leahy, M. M. (2010). Uniqueness and individuality in stuttering therapy. In A. L. Weiss (ed.), *Perspectives on Individual Differences Affecting Therapeutic Change in Communication Disorders*. London: Psychological Press.

Stewart, T. & Richardson, G. (2004). A qualitative study of therapeutic effect from a user's perspective. *Journal of Fluency Disorders*. 29, 95–108. 10.1016/j.jfludis.2003.11.001

Turnbull, J. (2000). The transtheoretical model of change: examples from stammering. *Counselling Psychology Quarterly*. 31 (1), 13–21. 10.1080/09515070050011033

Turnbull, J. & Stewart, T. (2010). *The Dysfluency Resource Book*. London: Routledge.

3 Considering Commonalities in Stuttering Therapy

Kurt Eggers, Sharon K. Millard, and J. Scott Yaruss

Introduction

There has been much discussion within our field about whether one treatment approach is somehow better than another approach. For example, there have been differences of opinion about so-called 'stutter-more-fluently' versus 'speak-more-fluently' approaches with teens and adults, counselling versus direct speech work, and indirect versus direct approaches with young children. Underpinning all of these discussions is the assumption that one therapy is or will be, more effective than another. In this chapter, we propose that, the quest for the 'best therapy' is unlikely to provide us with the knowledge we seek. Instead, we suggest that it is better to ask ourselves why a treatment approach is effective and why certain approaches appear to be more effective with particular clients.

In their systematic review, Baxter et al. (2015) concluded that even though there has been much research into stuttering treatment efficacy and effectiveness, there is no evidence that one programme yields better results than another. In this chapter, we argue that this might be explained by the contextual model, which suggests that it is the similarities between treatment approaches, rather than the differences, that which account for successful outcomes. We will use programmes that are currently researched and widely available for treating young children who stutter to provide examples of why this view may be applicable in our field. Finally, we will conclude with some important implications for both researchers and clinicians.

The Contextual Model

A medical model perspective is often used to explain why something works in treatment, where specific treatment techniques or methods are regarded as the reason for change. This medical model has been the centre of debate because in the field of clinical psychology, the treatment itself was found to account for little outcome variance. While a series of meta-analyses showed that therapy is better than no therapy, to the surprise of many researchers,

DOI: 10.4324/9781003179016-3

they also showed that one approach does not lead to a significantly better outcome than another (Wampold, 2015).

With rare exception, research has uncovered little significant difference among different psychotherapeutic approaches, an observation that has been described as "the dodo effect". Herder et al. (2006) found similar results in a meta-analysis of behavioural treatments for stuttering. Their results support the claim that intervention for stuttering results in an overall positive effect, but also show that no one treatment approach demonstrates significantly greater effects over another treatment approach.

Although specific techniques or methods were not found to be associated with the success of psychological treatment, Wampold (2015) did identify four specific factors that are common across a variety of treatment approaches; these factors account for much of the variance in treatment outcome. These "common" or "therapeutic" factors that facilitate and sustain change are: (a) the nature of the working alliance formed between the client and the clinician (e.g., emotional bonding, shared goal-setting, agreement on methods); (b) the characteristics of the client and his/her environment (e.g., temperament, family support); (c) the client's and the clinician's hopefulness that change can happen (e.g., belief that treatment will work); and (d) the specific treatment techniques (in stuttering treatment, these may include desensitisation or easy onsets, etc.). Wampold et al. have argued that the first three factors contribute more to outcome of treatment than the specific techniques used.

The contextual model, a relationship model based on these common factors, states that there are three pathways through which treatment effects (i.e., symptom reduction and better quality of life) can be achieved (see Figure 3.1). These pathways or relationship factors integrate common factors and specific factors. Although some treatments may emphasise one pathway over another, to be optimally effective, any treatment should utilise all three pathways (Wampold, 2017). The first pathway is based on the fact that an understanding relationship between an empathic and caring clinician and clients and their environment adds to the client's well-being. Critical to the expectation pathway is that the client and client system genuinely believe that the

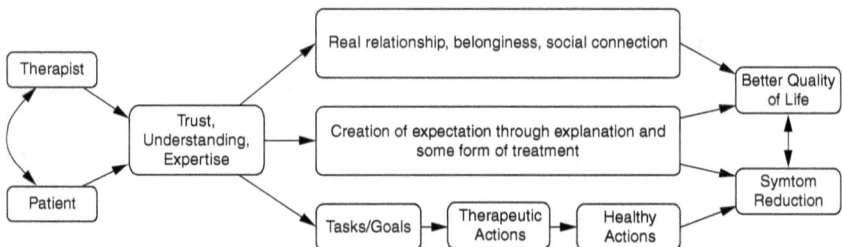

Figure 3.1 The contextual model (Wampold & Imel, 2015).

explanations provided by the clinician about the disorder and the related treatment actions will result in addressing the problem. This also entails that the clinician and the client (system) need to agree on treatment goals and specific treatment actions, two critical components of therapeutic alliance. Finally, the contextual model states that specific therapeutic actions (third pathway) with clearly structured (sub)goals not only create certain expectations but also result in changes remediating existing problems.

Several components of this contextual model have been studied in the stuttering field. For example, the importance of a trusting therapeutic alliance was documented both in adults who stutter (Sønsterud et al., 2019) and in young children who stutter (Coleman & Kaplan, 1990). Limited understanding of the clinical process or a mismatch between child and family expectations resulted in a poor therapeutic alliance and a higher risk for dropping out of therapy. Children and their families were also found to respond more positively to treatment when informed about various topics, including the nature and aetiology of stuttering, the content and structure of therapy, specific roles for the client and clinician, and expected outcomes from intervention.

Could This Contextual Model Be Relevant and Applicable to Stuttering Therapy?

A number of therapies and approaches are recommended for stuttering across the lifespan, with differing levels of empirical evidence to support them (Baxter et al., 2015; Brignell et al., 2021). The programmes that are most well-known and widely available for clinicians to study, and those with the greatest amount of efficacy and effectiveness research, are focused on young children. In order to consider the potential relevance of the contextual model, we have selected four of these programmes as a basis for discussion. The published details of each should be explored further by the reader; the summaries below highlight the main features:

The Lidcombe Program (LP; Onslow et al., 2020)

Theoretical underpinning: stuttering is a behaviour that can be reduced through operant conditioning principles.

Aim: For young children who stutter to achieve no stuttering or almost no stuttering.

Methods: Parents are taught to provide 'verbal contingencies' to their children's speech, beginning in structured practice sessions and then in conversation. When children are fluent, parents praise and request self-evaluation and/or acknowledge fluent speech. When children stutter, parents may acknowledge the stuttering or request that the child self-corrects. There should be substantially more praise for fluency than requests for self-correction. Parents collect daily severity ratings, and when the child achieves zero or little stuttering they enter a maintenance phase.

Evidence: Children who receive the LP show significantly reduced stuttering frequency compared to those who do not and the intervention is as effective when delivered in groups and via telehealth (see Brignell et al., 2021 for review).

RESTART-Demands and Capacities Model (RESTART-DCM; Franken & Laroes, 2021)

Theoretical underpinning: Stuttering is a consequence of a mismatch between the demands and capacities that a child experiences at each moment in time.

Aim: To decrease demands in the environment and increase the child's capacities for speaking fluently, creating a balance that results in fluent speech (de Sonneville-Koedoot et al., 2015).

Methods: A multifactorial assessment is conducted to identify the child's capacities for fluent speech and the communication demands placed on them. In Step 1, parents are taught, through observation of the clinician, to reduce linguistic and emotional demands so that they match the child's capacities for fluency. Parents change their interaction style, firstly during clinic sessions and then at home during Special Times. In Step 2 (if necessary) the focus is on increasing speech motor, language, and emotional capacities. A small proportion of children go to Step 3, when they are taught strategies to modify the moment of stuttering and increase tolerance to stuttering.

Evidence: RESTART-DCM is as effective and as cost-effective as the LP (de Sonneville-Koedoot et al., 2015) across a range of outcomes (including stuttering frequency, speech attitude, and quality of life), with a similar number of sessions for each (mean 22 and 19 for LP and RESTART-DCM respectively).

Palin Parent–Child Interaction Therapy (Palin PCI; Kelman & Nicholas, 2020)

Theoretical underpinning: Stuttering is a multifactorial condition, with physiological, linguistic, emotional, and environmental factors interacting with the genetic predisposition to stutter.

Aims: To reduce stuttering frequency and/or struggle; to reduce the impact of the stuttering on child and parents; to increase parents' knowledge of stuttering and confidence in how to support their child.

Methods: A comprehensive assessment is conducted to identify factors that influence fluency, stuttering, and confident communication. Therapy is made up of Interaction, Family, and Child Strategies. Parents first identify interaction strategies that are relevant for their child through video–observation of parent-child interaction, then practise these in 5-minute play sessions (Special Time) at home. The more indirect components (Interaction and Family strategies) are introduced over six therapy sessions, with more direct Child Strategies introduced if necessary afterwards.

Evidence: The therapy is effective in reducing stuttering frequency and impact, as well as increasing parents' knowledge and confidence to support their children. Benefits are maintained for up to one year post therapy (Millard et al., 2008; 2009; 2018).

Comprehensive/Family-focused Treatment Approach (Yaruss & Reeves, 2017)

Theoretical underpinning: Stuttering is the result of the interaction of child factors, interpersonal stressors, and environmental stressors, influenced by underlying genetic and neurological differences.

Aims: To provide parents with counseling and support; to support the development of easier speech; and to develop healthy attitudes to stuttering in both parent and child.

Methods: There are three elements within this programme: 1) In parent-focused treatment, parents are educated about stuttering, how to reduce communicative stressors, and how to establish an environment that supports the child's ease of speaking 2) Parent and child understanding and acceptance of stuttering is addressed through counselling, education, and desensitisation to stuttering. These less-direct components provide the foundations for 3) direct child communication modifications, if needed, which include speech modification, stuttering modification, and communication skills development.

Evidence: Children demonstrated a significant reduction in stuttering frequency post treatment which was maintained over time, with a mean number of 12 sessions. Parents rated high levels of satisfaction with the programme (Yaruss et al., 2006).

Differences in the Approaches

Programmes are described and taught with an emphasis on features that the authors consider to be important and which make each programme identifiable and distinct from others. Treatment fidelity (how closely the clinician adheres to the programmes principles and methods) is emphasised within the research and is considered to be critical. Once the efficacy and effectiveness of an intervention has been established, the next stage in the research process is to explore the critical components of the therapy, a stage that only the LP researchers have achieved thus far. Unsurprisingly, the critical components are assumed to be those that are the key characteristics of the programme that set it apart from others.

Certainly, there are differences between these approaches, e.g., in their theoretical perspectives. While the LP considers stuttering within a behavioural framework, others programmes take a more multifactorial view of stuttering. This requires a more comprehensive assessment process and a more flexible approach to the content of the therapy.

The goals of the approaches also differ. The LP seeks to eliminate or reduce stuttering to a low level. Both RESTART-DCM and the LP continue until 'acceptable fluency levels' are reached. Palin PCI and the Comprehensive Approach seek to reduce struggling and increase fluency, but there is a greater emphasis on communication and participation. A reduction in stuttering *impact* is considered critical for successful outcome, both for parents and children, in these two approaches, and the importance of addressing the needs of parents is explicit and evaluated as part of therapy outcome.

The methods have their origins in differing counselling methods, including operant conditioning, behaviour modification, family systems therapies, strengths versus deficit-focused approaches, and Cognitive Behaviour Therapy. How parents are supported differs in style, with parents being 'taught', 'instructed', 'shown' or 'facilitated to find their own' targets within therapy. Palin PCI is notable in its inclusion of both parents in therapy being usual practice.

Regarding direct work on speech production: in the LP, "children are not instructed to change their customary speech pattern in any way;" however, in the other programmes, the changes that children make are explicit. Activities for desensitisation and acceptance of stuttering are explicitly included in both Palin PCI and the Comprehensive Approach, and the value of the therapy for developing skills to manage stuttering are discussed throughout.

Similarities in the Approaches

Although it is true that numerous differences can be identified in the various treatment approaches as reviewed above, it is also true that similarities exist. These similarities are in the goals of the treatments, the methods employed to achieve those goals, the adaptations that clinicians are taught to make to ensure the success of treatment, and also in the measured outcomes and demonstrated efficacy of the treatments. For example, we have noted that the approaches described above differ in the degree to which they emphasise increased fluency and decreased stuttering in the broader context of effective communication. Still, the fact remains that all of the approaches do address these aspects of speech production, either as primary goals or as part of a broader set of desired outcomes. This is not surprising, given that an overarching purpose of therapies for early childhood stuttering is to alleviate stuttering and the problems that may be associated with stuttering. What is notable, however, is that all four programmes highlighted take as a fundamental assumption the notion that it *is* possible for children to increase their fluency and improve their communication and that it is possible to achieve positive change through intervention. None of the programmes automatically presume that a young child who stutters will necessarily continue to do so into adulthood, and all of the programs presume that therapy can be beneficial for the child and the parents.

In addition to starting with the assumption that change in children's fluency *is* possible, all four programmes favour early intervention instead of taking a "wait and see" approach to determining the appropriate timing for therapy. The approaches may differ in terms of the specific triggers that they use for determining that the time is right to initiate therapy (e.g., assessment of "risk factors"). Still, none of the four approaches advocate lengthy periods of observation or waiting to see if a child happens to "outgrow" stuttering on their own, as was once the case, and all four emphasise the importance of accounting for parental concerns in deciding in favour of treatment. These programmes also prefer early intervention in an attempt to prevent the development of chronic stuttering and/or the potential long-term consequences of stuttering and to ensure that the child and parents are supported as the child's fluency development unfolds over time.

Even more to the point, the treatments all share similarities in how they go about achieving their goals of improved speech fluency and communication. For example, all of the treatments are founded on significant involvement of the parents. In fact, all of the treatments are essentially parent-administered, at least in the early stages. Though what the programmes ask or teach parents to do may differ based on the orientation the programmes hold toward the nature of stuttering, they still all have significant parent training and counselling components. This is particularly seen in Palin PCI, Restart-DCM, and the Comprehensive Approach, each of which devote extensive time and effort to helping parents learn about stuttering and the factors that may affect their child's speech fluency and communication as a whole. These programmes also involve ample attention to exploring parents' own feelings and attitudes toward stuttering and to helping parents come to terms with their fears and concerns about their child's present and future stuttering. The programmes also rely on this parent foundation to support the child's own development of positive communication attitudes, so that the child will continue to speak freely and without fear even if the stuttering should persist. Clearly, the LP approaches parent involvement differently. There, the focus is on helping parents learn to provide contingencies in the appropriate fashion and on the correct schedule (although recent research has questioned the necessity of such contingencies; see Donaghy et al., 2020). Still, the fact that parent participation is fundamental to the treatment highlights the fact that parent involvement and time spent focused on talking and communication with the child is a consistent, common factor in a range of different early childhood stuttering therapy approaches.

Another key similarity – and one that stands out in light of historical views about stuttering therapy for young children – is the fact that all four approaches highlighted in this paper directly acknowledge, discuss, and address stuttering with both the parents and children at some point in the therapy process. In the LP, for example, parents are taught early in therapy to identify moments of stuttered versus fluent speech, so that they can provide appropriate contingencies. In the Comprehensive Approach, parents are taught to acknowledge moments of stuttering in a supportive and open way, directly letting the child know that stuttering is nothing to be afraid of or ashamed of. Parents are taught to provide similar supportive comments as appropriate in the other approaches, as well. This is notable, because such direct discussion of stuttering would not have been favoured in so-called "indirect" therapy approaches that were common in the later portion of the 20th century. Again, the specific messages provided to children by parents differ depending upon the programme: LP involves praise for fluency whereas other programmes may involve praise for communication attempts, regardless of whether or not they appear to contain stuttering. Still, none of the approaches shy away from addressing speaking or stuttering directly, as needed, thereby highlighting the now-common, but once less-accepted belief, that it is okay to talk about stuttering with young children.

Further commonalities can be seen in the everyday application of the treatments: e.g., all of these approaches highlight the importance of individualising treatments for each unique child's and family's needs. In addition, each approach involves making changes to the child's communication environment (whether in the short term or long term) in order to increase the likelihood that the child will produce more fluent speech. This latter point is interesting, because changes in communication environment are explicitly included in the Palin PCI, RESTART-DCM, and Comprehensive Approach. In apparent contrast, earlier writings about the LP excluded changing the child's linguistic context to enhance fluency; however, more recent writing has shown that clinicians may indeed make changes to the child's communication environment (e.g., the use of closed or binary questions, language contingent with the situation, and the impact of the choice of toy, all possible areas of focus in the more indirect components of other therapies) in order to elicit more fluent speech which can then be reinforced via appropriate contingencies (Onslow et al., 2021).

Another key commonality across approaches is one that matches what has been learned from studies of the commonalities in various psychotherapeutic and counselling approaches: all four approaches described involve the development of a therapeutic alliance between the parents and the clinician and, as more-direct aspects of therapy are incorporated, between the child and the clinician. Fostering this therapeutic alliance involves building a supportive relationship between client and clinician; one in which the client feels comfortable sharing their fears and concerns while the clinician provides understanding, validation, support, and, as needed, guidance. Again, the ways in which this alliance are accomplished differ depending upon the specific approach, but relationship-building is still at the heart of the clinical interaction. For example, the Palin PCI, RESTART-DCM, and Comprehensive Approach explicitly focus on identifying the needs of parents (and, again as needed, children themselves) for counselling and support. This is accomplished through various counselling strategies including scaling activities, guided interviewing, and discussions about hopes and dreams for the child. Although the LP appears to focus more on educating parents about the steps involved in providing contingencies, it is clear that parents still develop a trusting relationship with their clinician, who provides a sounding board and guide as the parent seeks to learn how to support their child's speech production. As shown in common factors research outside of our field, the therapeutic alliance is the factor that contributes most to the positive changes associated with therapy, so the development of this relationship in these therapy approaches is particularly important and relevant for our consideration of commonalities across approaches.

What Does This Mean for Clinicians and Researchers?

The empirical evidence and the understanding of factors that contribute to successful outcomes within the Contextual Model suggest that any of these therapies has potential to be 'successful' for an individual child who stutters. The Contextual Model would suggest that the clinician should pay particular attention to factors that are similar across the programmes to maximise outcomes. All the therapies emphasise the need for training; the Contextual Model also highlights the need for clinicians to be knowledgeable and have confidence in the approach they are using. Having a strong rationale, experience in using a programme, and the belief that it will be helpful for the client are linked to improved outcomes. Therefore, proper training in one approach that fits a clinician's philosophical perspective is the first step.

Working with parents is a clear similarity across the therapies, so any intervention with this population should involve parents as key participants in the process. Parents are involved to deliver the therapy and support the child *and* to address their own needs, worries, and confidence. Reinforcing the parent-child relationship, encouraging openness in the family, and fostering a positive attitude to stuttering will also be key.

Working with families to foster a positive therapeutic relationship is critical. Clinicians can help parents understand and believe in what they are doing by developing shared and realistic goals modified and adapted according to the child's need, temperament, and response to treatment; helping parents explore and understand the rationale for the goals and methods; and providing a learning environment that is supportive, motivating, and reinforcing will facilitate child and parent engagement and help parents become increasingly less reliant on the clinician.

Conclusion

The most important message to take away from this review is that there is choice: choice for clinicians in terms of which approach they are educated to practise in and use, and choice for parents about which therapy they think will best meet the needs of their family. This does not mean that whatever a clinician might do will necessarily work. Method and procedure are still important, but regardless of the method or procedure, a strong therapeutic alliance is a prerequisite for therapy. Clients and parents need to be informed about the nature and the aetiology of stuttering, as well as the specific treatment goals and actions involved in the treatment. In addition, they need to be cogently guided through the different treatment steps. When one approach is not having the expected or desired effect, there are options to consider. In the future, we may have better data to help us determine whether one approach will be better than another for an individual child. At present, we can be confident in the knowledge that we can help children communicate with greater confidence and more ease while also meeting the needs of parents, and we should not expect to achieve this in just one way.

References

Baxter, S., Johnson, M., Blank, L., Cantrell, A., Brumfitt, S., Enderby, P., & Goyder, E. (2015). The state of the art in non-pharmacological interventions for developmental stuttering. Part 1: a systematic review of effectiveness. *International journal of language & communication disorders.* 50 (5), 676–718. 10.1111/1460-6984.12171

Brignell, A., Krahe, M., Downes, M., Kefalianos, E., Reilly, S., & Morgan, A. (2021). Interventions for children and adolescence who stutter: A systematic review, meta-analysis, and evidence map. *Journal of Fluency Disorders.* 105843. 10.1016/j.jfludis.2021.105843

Coleman, D. & Kaplan, M. (1990). Effects of pretherapy video preparation on child therapy outcomes. *Professional Psychology: Research and Practice.* 21 (3), 199–203. 10.1037/0735-7028.21.3.199

de Sonneville-Koedoot, C., Stolk, E., Rietveld, T., & Franken, M. C. (2015). Direct versus indirect treatment for preschool children who stutter: The RESTART randomized trial. *PloS one.* 10 (7), e0133758. 10.1371/journal.pone.0133758

Donaghy, M., O'Brian, S., Onslow, M., Lowe, R., Jones, M., & Menzies, R. G. (2020). Verbal Contingencies in the Lidcombe Program: A Noninferiority Trial. *Journal of Speech, Language, and Hearing Research.* 63 (October), 1–13. 10.1044/2020_jslhr-20-00155

Franken, M. C., & Laroes, E. (2021). RESTART-DCM Method. Revised edition 2021. https://www.restartdcm.nl

Herder, C., Howard, C., Nye, C., & Vanryckeghem, M. (2006). Effectiveness of behavioral stuttering treatment: A Systemic Review and Meta-Analysis. *Contemporary Issues in Communication Science and Disorders.* 33, 61–73. 10.1044/cicsd_33_S_61

Kelman, E., & Nicholas, A. (2020) *Palin Parent-Child Interaction Therapy for Early Childhood Stammering* (2nd Edition). London: Routledge. 10.4324/9781351122351

Millard, S. K., Edwards, S., & Cook, F. M. (2009). Parent-child interaction therapy: Adding to the evidence. *International Journal of Speech-Language Pathology.* 11 (1), 61–76. 10.1080/17549500802603895

Millard, S. K., Nicholas A., & Cook F. M. (2008). Is parent-child interaction therapy effective in reducing stuttering? *Journal of Speech, Language and Hearing Research.* 51 (3), 636–650. 10.1044/1092-4388(2008/046)

Millard, S. K., Zebrowski, P., & Kelman, E. (2018). Palin parent–child interaction therapy: The bigger picture. *American journal of speech-language pathology.* 27 (3S), 1211–1223. 10.1044/2018_AJSLP-ODC11-17-0199

Onslow, M., Webbeter, M., Harrison, E., Arnott, S., Bridgman, K., Carey, B., Sheedy, S., O'Brian, S., MacMillan, V., Lloyd, W., & Hearne, A. (2021, December 6). The

Lidcombe Program treatment guide. Retrieved from https://www.uts.edu.au/sites/default/files/2021-04/Lidcombe%20Program%20Treatment%20Guide%202021%20v1.3%202021-04-27.pdf

Onslow, M., Webber, M., Harrison, E., Arnott, S., Bridgman, K., Carey, B., Sheedy, S., O'Brian, S., MacMillan, V., Lloyd, W., & Hearne, A. (2020). *The Lidcombe Program Treatment Guide November 2020 (Version 1.1)*. Downloaded from https://www.uts.edu.au/sites/default/files/2020-12/Lidcombe%20Program%20Treatment%20Guide%202020%20v1.1%202020-12-07_1.pdf

Sønsterud, H., Kirmess, M., Howells, K., Ward, D., Feragen, K. B., & Halvorsen, M. S. (2019). The working alliance in stuttering treatment: a neglected variable? *International Journal of Language and Communication Disorders*. 54, 606–619. 10.1111/1460-6984.12465

Wampold B. E. (2015). How important are the common factors in psychotherapy? An update. *World psychiatry*. 14 (3), 270–277. 10.1002/wps.20238

Wampold, B. E. (2017). What should we practice?: A contextual model for how psychotherapy works. In T. Rousmaniere, R. K. Goodyear, S. D. Miller, & B. E. Wampold (Eds.), *The cycle of excellence: Using deliberate practice to improve supervision and training* (pp. 49–65). Wiley-Blackwell. 10.1002/9781119165590.ch3

Wampold, B. E., & Imel, Z. E. (2015). *The great psychotherapy debate: The evidence for what makes psychotherapy work*. (2nd ed.). New York, NY: Routledge Publications.

Yaruss, J. S., Coleman, C., & Hammer, D. (2006). Treating preschool children who stutter: Description and preliminary evaluation of a family-focused treatment approach. *Language, Speech, and Hearing Services in Schools*. 37, 118–136. 10.1044/0161-1461(2006/014)

Yaruss, J. S. & Reeves, N. (2017). *Early childhood stuttering therapy: A practical guide*. McKinney, TX: Stuttering Therapy Resources, Inc.

4 Children Showing Signs of Stuttering

Veerle Waelkens and Sabine Van Eerdenbrugh

Introduction

Accurately predicting recovery from stuttering in preschool children (below 6 years of age) with or without treatment is not yet possible. A large group of children recovers naturally from stuttering within 4 years after stuttering onset (Yairi & Ambrose, 1999). For a long time, waiting for natural recovery was the recommended approach. A preschool child who stutters, however, rarely recovers naturally within the first year after onset. One child (of 16 = 6.3%) recovered within the first 19.4 months after onset in a study of Carey et al. (2020) and five (of 84 = 6%) recovered in 12 to 17 months after onset without treatment or with minimal stuttering management advice in a study of Yairi and Ambrose (1999).

Waiting for natural recovery to occur is no longer the accepted approach and is even unethical. Reasons are a low natural recovery rate of preschool children who stutter in the first year after stuttering onset (Carey et al., 2020; Yairi & Ambrose, 1999), the increasing awareness of preschool children about their stuttering (e.g., Langevin et al., 2010; Vanryckeghem et al., 2005), the significant negative impact of stuttering on emotional, social and behavioural development and wellbeing throughout the life span (e.g., Briley & Ellis, 2020; McAllister, 2016) and the high treatment success rate in preschool children who stutter (e.g., de Sonneville-Koedoot et al., 2015; Jones et al., 2005). Instead of waiting for natural recovery, the clinician needs to decide about initiating treatment, not initiating treatment or perform other steps in the assessment procedure. Making such decisions is essential but may be difficult. The five cases in this chapter aim at facilitating this process of clinical reasoning.

Client Information

To explain the steps in the assessment procedure, we present five cases of preschool children who stuttered (retrospectively). We apply different reasoning processes to these cases depending on the needs of each child. The steps of the diagnostic assessment process are illustrated in Figure 4.1.

DOI: 10.4324/9781003179016-4

```
┌─────────────────────────┐
│      Step1: Initial     │
│  assessment of the child│
└─────────────────────────┘
            │
┌─────────────────────────┐
│   Step 2: Education about│
│  stuttering and addressing│
│   concerns of the child and│
│ family related to the stuttering│
└─────────────────────────┘
```

Step 3: General tips to reduce demands of communication at home (optional step)

Step 4: Active monitoring of the stuttering behaviour (optional step)

Step 5: Follow-up (always follows Step 3 and Step 4)

Step 6: Treatment or No treatment

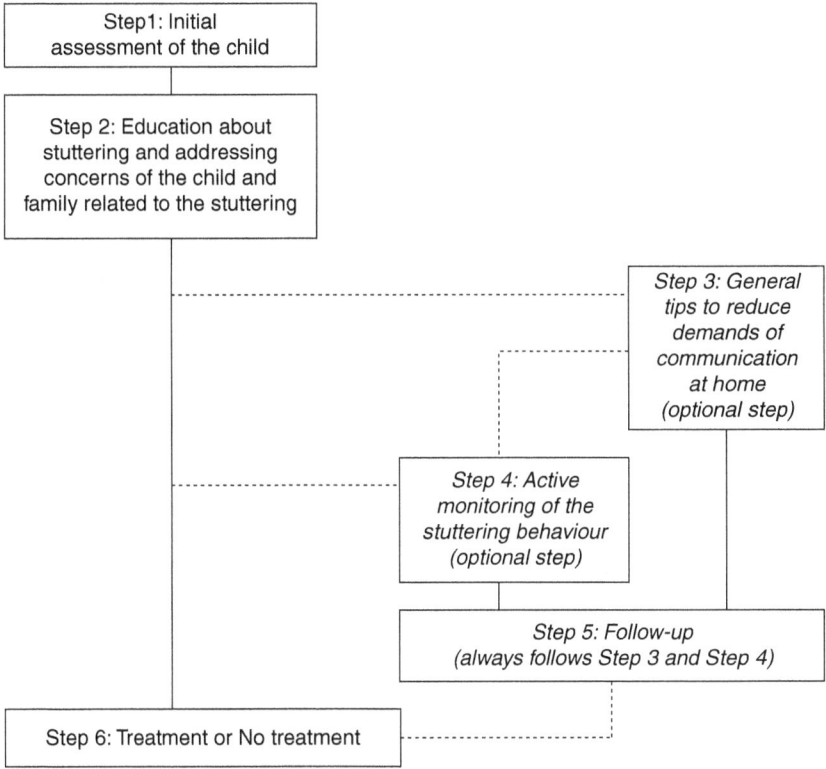

Dashed line = optional step; solid line = standard step; *text in italic* refers to steps before treatment

Figure 4.1 Six steps in the diagnostic assessment process.

During the initial assessment (Step 1), we collect general socio-demographic information, medical, family and treatment history, including motoric, linguistic, emotional and social development, milestones, communicative challenges and strengths and the status of the child's hearing. Detailed information about the stuttering (onset, types, frequency, development over time, reaction of the child and parents to the stuttering and so on) is also collected. Table 4.1 provides a concise summary of the clinical findings, collected during the initial assessment. The selection of information for Table 4.1 is based on the factors listed by Singer et al. (2020) that are related to persistence of stuttering in descending order of statistically significant effect size. Information about the development of stuttering since stuttering onset and the response of child and parent(s) to the stuttering is added to the table (Sugathan & Maruthy, 2020; Yairi & Ambrose, 2005) since this information was not included in the review of Singer et al. (2020).

Not surprisingly, as speech and language are in full development during preschool years, some of the children also experienced speech or language

Table 4.1 Information and clinical findings from the initial assessment

Risks for stuttering persistence	Preschool child 1	Preschool child 2	Preschool child 3	Preschool child 4	Preschool child 5
Family history of stuttering or recovery (present)[$]	Not present	Present (brother and father, recovered)	Not present	Not recovered (father)	Not present
Gender (male)[$]	Male	Female	Male	Male	Male
Age at onset (older)[$]	3;03	2;11	3;00	3;07	3;00
Speech sound skills (lower)[$,#]	Normal, a few phonological processes to be monitored (fronting and backing). The processes are always present in the speech	Normal, not measured	Normal, not measured	Normal, not measured	Two phonological processes still present, one not age-appropriate (fronting and cluster reduction)
Number of Stuttering-Like-Dysfluencies (SLD) (higher)[$,*]	Very mild stuttering, mostly OD	No stuttering during clinic sessions (at home: mainly OD)	Mild stuttering	Severe stuttering	Moderate stuttering
Receptive language (lower)[$]	Normal (CELF)	Advanced, not measured	Normal, not measured	Not measured	Native language normal, not measured – is acquiring a second language
Expressive language (lower)[$]	Normal (CELF), needs time	Advanced, not measured	Normal, (advanced according to the parents), not measured	Advanced, not measured	Native language normal, not measured – is acquiring a second language
Negative/positive reactivity (greater)[°]	Not measured	Not measured	Not measured	Not measured	Not measured

Family history of persistent stuttering (present)°	Not present	Not present	Not present	Father occasionally, in emotional situations	Not present
Number of individual SLD-types (higher)°,#	All SLD but no tension, not frequent	Mainly repetitions, not frequent	Repetitions and subtle (mild) blocks, not frequent	Repetitions, prolongations and blocks, frequent	Repetitions, prolongations, frequent
Expressive vocabulary (lower)°	Word-finding difficulties. CELF normal	Advanced, not measured	Normal, (advanced according to the parents), not measured	Advanced, not measured	Native language normal, not measured – is acquiring a second language
Number of SLD within 1 year of onset (stable or increasing)^,#	Periodically (not stable, not increasing)	Fluctuating (e.g., not during the clinic session)	Periodically (not stable, not increasing)	Increasing	Stable
Severity ratings by CLINICIANs and parents (stable or increasing)^	Periodically (not stable, not increasing)	Fluctuating (e.g., not during clinic session)	Periodically (not stable, not increasing)	Increasing	Stable
Occurrence of secondary movements (stable or increasing)^	Extremely mild secondary behaviour, not consistent or frequent	Not present	Extremely mild secondary behaviour, not consistent or frequent	Clearly present, not consistent or frequent	Mild secondary behaviour, stable, not frequent

(*Continued*)

Table 4.1 (Continued)

Risks for stuttering persistence	Preschool child 1	Preschool child 2	Preschool child 3	Preschool child 4	Preschool child 5
Time since onset (more than 1 year)^	8 months	1 month	3 months	1 month	12 months
Response of child/ parents to stuttering^	Is more silent at preschool than before	Is a verbal child but does not show negative reaction to the stuttering	Does not show negative reaction to the stuttering	Does not show negative reaction to the stuttering	Shows signs of frustration when blocking

Notes
$ = Sufficient evidence according to the review of Singer et al., 2020.
° = Insufficient evidence according to the review of Singer et al., 2020, but at least one study reported statistical significance.
^ = Evidence from the study of Yairi & Ambrose, 2005.
# = Evidence from the review of Sugathan & Murathy, 2020.
* OD = Other dysfluencies. SLD and OD were observed in a speech sample, using a Dutch test that corresponds with the SSI-4; underlined text: factors that indicate more risk for persistence of stuttering according to Singer et al., 2020, Sugathan & Murathy, 2020 and Yairi & Ambrose, 2005.

difficulties. It is not always necessary to administer a formal assessment for speech or language development for each preschool child who stutters. Only if a child shows signs of difficulty or doubts, they are reported.

Diagnostic Assessment

The diagnostic assessment starts with Step 1 (Figure 4.1), the initial assessment, and can take up to six steps. Step 2 is the education of the parents and the child. We include this step for all preschool children who stutter and their families. We discuss with the child and their parents what stuttering is, inform parents about persistence and recovery of stuttering, explain how stuttering may develop, identify with the parents the types and severity of the child's stuttering and address other stuttering-related concerns. These include reactions of the child, parents or others towards the stuttering (including teasing, mocking or bullying). This conversation takes place during the initial assessment with the child and the parents or with the parents alone at another time.

Step 3 is an optional step. It includes providing general tips (without training) such as asking parents to decrease the number of questions that they ask the child or to add more pauses during a conversation. This step is often not necessary. It depends on the family and child: some families do not set high demands on communicative situations and some children do not experience communicative demands as a trigger for stuttering.

Step 4, active monitoring, is also an optional step. Some children periodically produce dysfluencies (stuttering appears and disappears for days, weeks or months), some produce stuttering that is not stable or consistent (in some situations the stuttering occurs, in other similar situations it does not) and some produce very mild stuttering behaviour with mostly typical dysfluencies, also labelled as 'other dysfluencies' (OD). For two preschool children, we prefer to observe the stuttering behaviour for some time to gain insight in the development of the stuttering. Taking this step is justifiable, knowing that the children are well before the age of 6 years so that treatment can take place before that crucial age (e.g., de Sonneville-Koedoot et al., 2015; Jones et al., 2005) and knowing that the stuttering does not cause concern, frustration or any other negative feeling or reaction to the children nor the parents.

We train parents during the clinic session in how to report stuttering severity for daily conversations with the child in different and representative samples. The parent learns to identify stuttering moments, even when they are subtle or mild. This often takes more than one clinic session. The severity ratings (for example on a 10-point Likert scale) from the parents need to be reliable and accurate. Another tool can be used to record stuttering severity. It is, however, important that parents understand what stuttering is and that parents correctly identify the stuttering of their child. Parents record stuttering severity at a frequency that they agree on with the clinician (e.g., daily, every second day, three times a week) but it needs to be sufficiently frequent to allow correct interpretation.

After Step 3 or Step 4, we discuss with the parents the time interval for the next clinic visit (Step 5) to evaluate the implementation of the tips or the monitoring of the stuttering, e.g., every 4 weeks, every 6 weeks, every 2 months.

Step 6 is the final step of the diagnostic assessment. At that point, we initiate treatment or decide that treatment is not necessary.

Diagnostic Assessment Preschool Child 1

Clinical decision: We provide the parents and Child 1 with information about stuttering in case stuttering severity increases over time (Step 2). Step 3 seems a necessary step at this point in time for the child's family and for the teacher. We explain to them that communicative situations can be more demanding for some preschool children who stutter, and probably also for Child 1. We give tips to the parents to reduce language-loaded family situations. Because the stuttering behaviour is extremely mild, we do not include Step 4. A follow-up session (Step 5) is planned 3 months after the initial assessment. At this point in time, the situation of Child 1 is not indicating an immediate need for stuttering treatment as his behaviour at preschool is normalised and the stuttering severity is not increasing.

Clinical plan: Step 1 – Step 2 – Step 3 – Step 5.

Diagnostic Assessment Preschool Child 2

Clinical decision: We provide Child 2 and her parents with information about stuttering (Step 2). The motoric planning skills are most likely not synchronised with the advanced language development of Child 2. Hence, we decide to allow more time for speech and language to develop and to align to each other. We plan a follow-up session in 3 months' time (Step 5).

Clinical plan: Step 1 – Step 2 – Step 5.

Diagnostic Assessment Preschool Child 3

Clinical decision: After providing parents and Child 3 the information about stuttering (Step 2), we decide that it is not necessary yet to initiate stuttering treatment. The stuttering appears in cycles and is mild at this point. Child 3's sometimes advanced language behaviour probably triggers the stuttering. We help the parents reducing the language demands and suggest adding pauses in conversations and modelling occasional OD during their own speech in conversations with the child (Step 3). Because the stuttering also contains more severe types of stuttering (blocks), we feel it necessary to have a clear view on the development of the stuttering. We ask for daily recordings of the stuttering severity until the following clinic session using a 10-point Likert scale (0 = no stuttering, 1 = extremely mild stuttering and 9 = extremely severe stuttering) (Step 4). During the initial assessment session at the clinic, we teach the parents to identify stuttering behaviour. We ask them not to use judgemental or evaluative vocabulary when discussing the severity, so they do not increase awareness in the child. We plan a follow-up clinic session in 2 months' time (Step 5).

Clinical plan: Step 1 – Step 2 – Step 3 – Step 4 – Step 5.

Diagnostic Assessment Preschool Child 4

Clinical decision: After providing parents and Child 4 information and support for stuttering (Step 2), we decide starting stuttering treatment because of the severe stuttering and because of the inconveniences it causes, resulting in secondary behaviour (Step 6).

Clinical plan: Step 1 – Step 2 – Step 6 (Treatment).

Diagnostic Assessment Preschool Child 5

Clinical decision: After providing parents and Child 5 information and support for stuttering (Step 2), we decide to start phonology treatment to increase the intelligibility for some time. At this moment, this is the child's biggest concern. We decide to help the parents reducing language demands (Step 3). In addition to this, we ask the parents to daily record the stuttering severity using a 10-point scale (Step 4).

Given the age of Child 5, the time since onset, the crucial age of 6 years and the fact that stuttering treatment is a long-term treatment of at least 6 to 9 months followed by a follow-up period of several months to a year, we consider it necessary to start stuttering treatment after 3 months because there is no clear impact of phonology treatment and of reducing the demands in conversations (Step 6). We stop the phonology treatment and start stuttering treatment.

We depend heavily on the parents for both treatments (phonology and stuttering) to succeed as we are limited to working directly with Child 5 (insufficient language acquisition in Dutch). We coach the parents to implement the treatments at home. Both treatments occur mainly in the native language of the child. When we work directly with him during the clinic sessions, we are using the limited amount of Dutch Child 5 has at that moment.

Clinical plan: Step 1 – Step 2 – Step 3 – Step 4 – Step 6 (Treatment).

Discussion

To decide if a preschool child who stutters would benefit from stuttering treatment, several factors need to be considered. The factors in Table 4.1 appear in order of significant statistical effect size, but from the five cases it becomes clear that they are not interpreted in that order in the clinical practice. For example, gender would not matter to us in the decision to treat or not to treat. The preschool child's speech (stuttering) can be sufficient to indicate the need for treatment. Sometimes, no other factors are necessary to convince us to initiate stuttering treatment. Other factors, such as an increasing severity or an increasing time since onset often play a more prominent role in the clinical decision-making process because with the more severe overt stuttering behaviour also negative emotions and thoughts related to the stuttering may develop. The two factors listed above, however, are not listed by Singer et al. (2020) as statistically significant to estimate the chance on stuttering persistence or stuttering recovery. Yairi and Ambrose (2005) listed these latter factors (development of the stuttering behaviour over time and response of the children and the parents to the stuttering) as important clinical factors. They are indeed helpful to make the decision. For the cases in this chapter, Child 4 shows stable stuttering behaviour and Child 5 presents an increasing number of stuttering moments. For both preschool children, we initiate stuttering treatment. Child 1 and Child 3 show periodical stuttering and for Child 2 the stuttering fluctuates according to the situation. For these three children, this is an important factor to decide to take steps other than introducing stuttering treatment immediately. Based on our clinical experience, we rank these factors for preschool children who stutter in order of clinical relevancy (see Table 4.2).

It is important to realise that these factors are often not sufficient by themself to make decisions about the need for stuttering treatment at the time of the initial assessment. It is rather the interaction of several factors that contribute to this decision. For example, if the time since onset is only 1 month, but the child is 5 years old at onset, we would be more likely to decide on introducing stuttering treatment. Or if the stuttering behaviour is severe, parents and child are concerned, but the stuttering is not (yet) stable or is not increasing, we might decide to initiate stuttering treatment if providing information about stuttering (Step 2) does not sufficiently change the level of concern. The impact of the stuttering behaviour on the child and the family would be too great to be left untreated.

Table 4.2 Clinically relevant factors, in descending order, to decide to start treatment immediately according to the authors' clinical expertise

Clinically relevant factor
1. Age at the time of onset
2. Time since onset
3. Stuttering development since onset (periodically or continuous, increasing or stable)
4. Severity of overt types, secondary behaviour) and covert stuttering (awareness, frustration, secondary behaviour, temperamental impact,…)
5. Family history (persistence/recovery of stuttering)
6. Reaction parents/family/teacher to the stuttering (knowledge about stuttering, verbal and non-verbal responses, level of concern,…)
7. Concomitant disorders (related to communication)
8. Treatment history

Besides these factors related to stuttering behaviour, a profound knowledge of the speech and language development of preschool children is crucial to correctly understand the entire context of a preschool child who stutters. The prevalence of speech sound disorders, referring to both articulation and phonological disorders, is reported between 3.4% to 9% in 4- to 8-year-old children (e.g., Eadie et al., 2014). The variability originates from different age groups and different methods applied to identify speech sound disorders. Eadie et al. (2014) reported a 3.6% incidence at the age of 4, with a male/female gender ratio of about 1/1.

Language impairments were reported in 7.4% of 5- to 6-year-old children (Tomblin et al., 1997) and in 13% of 4– to 5-year-old children (McLeod & Harrison, 2009), with a male/female gender ratio of about 4/3.

Speech and language impairments clearly occur in many preschool children. Children at this age acquire many new skills due to extensive neurological plasticity (Johnston, 2004; Stiles, 2000). Sometimes speech and language develop at a slower pace in one preschool child than another. Extra stimulation, maturation or speech or language treatment may overcome some speech and language difficulties. Lower incidence numbers for speech sound disorders and language disorders reported for older children confirm this assumption. Therefore, providing parents with tips to reduce language demands in communicative situations may resolve some difficulties that preschool children encounter.

Stuttering typically appears during preschool years (3 to 5 years) (Yairi & Ambrose, 1999). Knowing that the incidence numbers of speech sound disorders and language disorders at this age are reported between 3.6% and 13%, it is not surprising to note that many preschool children who stutter have concomitant speech or language disorders or difficulties beside their stuttering. Arndt and Healy (2001) questioned 241 clinicians from the US about concomitant disorders of 467 preschool children who stutter between 6 and 12 years of age and found that 44% presented with concomitant speech or language difficulties. Blood et al. (2003) found this in 62.8% of 2628 preschool children who stutter between 5 and 18 years of age. It is, however, equally important to realise that these two studies rely on reports of clinicians who were questioned about their caseloads. This may be an overestimation, as Nippold (2004) found that clinicians are more likely to recommend stuttering treatment to preschool children who stutter with concomitant disorders compared to preschool children who stutter without concomitant disorders.

Conclusion

To make the clinical decision to initiate stuttering treatment or not for preschool children who stutter, several factors need to be considered. The factors reported in research do not correspond one-on-one with the clinically relevant factors that are suggest by the authors of this chapter. Factors related to stuttering onset, development of the stuttering behaviour, severity of the overt and covert stuttering, age of the preschool children who stutter and family history of stuttering are factors that are most frequently considered to be clinically relevant in the decision if a preschool child needs stuttering treatment or not. It is crucial that clinicians also possess profound knowledge about typical speech and language development in preschool children besides profound knowledge of developmental stuttering, also. Only then can a clinician understand the appropriate context of a preschool child who stutters and introduce appropriate steps into the diagnostic assessment procedure and treatment.

References

Arndt, J. & Healy, E. C. (2001). Concomitant disorders in school-age children who stutter. *Language, Speech, and Hearing Services on Schools.* 32 (2), 68–78. 10.1044/0161-1461 (2001/006)

Blood, G. W., Ridenour, V. J., Qualls, C. D., & Hammer, C. S. (2003). Co-occurring disorders in children who stutter. *Journal of Communication Disorders.* 36 (6), 427–448. 10.1016/s0021-9924(03)00023-6

Briley, P. M. & Ellis, C. (2020). Behavioral, social, and emotional well-being in children who stutter: The influence of race-ethnicity. *Logopedics Phoniatrics Vocology*, 1–9. 10.1080/14015439.2020.1801833

Carey, B., Onslow, M., & O'Brian, S. (2020). Natural recovery from stuttering for a clinical cohort of pre-school children who received no treatment. *International Journal of Speech-Language Pathology*, 1–9. 10.1080/17549507.2020.1746399

de Sonneville-Koedoot, C., Stolk, E., Rietveld, T., & Franken. M. C. (2015). Direct versus indirect treatment for preschool children who stutter: The restart randomized trial. *PLoSONE.* 10 (7), E0133758. 10.1371/journal.pone.0133758

Eadie, P. et al., (2014) Speech sound disorder at 4 years: Prevalence, comorbidities, and predictors in a community cohort of children. *Developmental Medicine & Child Neurology.* 57 (6), pp. 578–584. Available at: 10.1111/dmcn.12635

Johnston, M. V. (2004). Clinical disorders of brain plasticity. *Brain and Development.* 26 (2), 73–80. 10.1016/s0387-7604(03)00102-5

Jones, M., Onslow, M., Packman, A., Williams, S., Ormond, T., Schwarz, I., & Gebski, V. (2005). Randomised controlled trial of the Lidcombe program of early stuttering intervention. *British Medical Journal.* 331 (7518), 659–661. 10.1136/bmj. 38520.451840.E0

Langevin, M., Packman, A., & Onslow, M. (2010). Parent perceptions of the impact of stuttering on their preschoolers and themselves. *Journal of Communications Disorders.* 43 (5), 407–423. 10.1016/j.jcomdis.2010.05.003

McAllister, J. (2016). Behavioural, emotional, and social development of children who stutter. *Journal of Fluency Disorders.* 50, 23–32. 10.1016/j.jfludis.2016.09.003

McLeod, S. & Harrison, L. J., 2009. Epidemiology of speech and language impairment in a nationally representative sample of 4- to 5-year-old children. *Journal of Speech, Language, and Hearing Research.* 52 (5), 1213–1229. 10.1044/1092-4388(2009/08-0085)

Nippold, M. A. (2004). Phonological and language disorders in children who stutter: impact on treatment recommendations. Clinical Linguistics & Phonetics, 18 (2), 145–159. 10.1080/02699200310001659070

Singer, C. M., Hessling, A., Kelly, E. M., Singer, L., & Jones, R. M. (2020). Clinical characteristics associated with stuttering persistence: A meta-analysis. *Journal of Speech, Language, and Hearing Research.* 63 (9). 2995–3018. 10.1044/2020_JSLHR-20-00096

Stiles, J. (2000). Neuroplasticity and cognitive development. *Developmental Neuropsychology.* 18 (2), 237–272.

Sugathan, N. & Maruthy, S. (2020). Predictive factors for persistence and recovery of stuttering in children: A systematic review. *International Journal of Speech-Language Pathology.* 1–13. 10.1080/17549507.2020.1812718

Tomblin, J. B., Records, N. L., Buckwalter, P., Zhang, x., Smith, E., & O'Brien, M. (1997). Prevalence of specific language impairment in kindergarten children. *Journal of speech, language, and Hearing Research.* 40 (6), 1245–1260.

Vanryckeghem, M., Brutten, G. J., & Hernandez, L. M. (2005). A comparatice investigation of the speech-associated attitude of preschool and kindergarten children who do and do not stutter. *Journal of Fluency Disorders.* 3 (4), 307–318. 10.1016/jfludis.2005.09.003

Yairi, E., & Ambrose, N. G. (1999). Early childhood stuttering I: persistency and recovery rates. *Journal of Speech Language and Hearing Research.* 42 (5), 1097. 10.1044/jslhr.4205.1097

Yairi, E., & Ambrose, N. G. (2005). *Early Childhood Stuttering.* Austin, TX: Pro-Ed.

5   Building Resilience in Children Who Stutter through Camp Dream. Speak. Live

Courtney Byrd, Mary O'Dwyer, and Kurt Eggers

Introduction

For most children who stutter worldwide, standard practice targets learning to reduce stuttering as one of the primary goals. Yet, many children will continue to stutter, despite years of trying not to do so. The immediate and long-term effects of fluency conformity during the school-age years are not trivial. A large amount of data indicates that preschool, school-age, and adolescents who stutter report negative attitudes toward communication. Their rejection of the way they talk causes them to engage in unhealthy coping strategies (e.g., social avoidance, rejection of social networks, reduced social activity) that exclude them from protective mechanisms known to improve quality of life (e.g., peer and familial support). Years later, after many failed attempts at fluency, many adults lament how different their lives would have been if only, as a child they could have been taught that it is truly ok to stutter (e.g., O'Dwyer et al., 2018).

The purpose of the present chapter is to review the theoretical framework, and participant outcomes of Camp Dream. Speak. Live. (Camp DSL), an intensive treatment program for children who stutter that focuses exclusively on the cognitive and affective components of stuttering. Despite the absent fluency focus, the substantial gains in communication that participants in this unique program experience, directly contribute to reduced stuttering and/or reduced fear of stuttering as a natural by-product of participation. Further, their gains are not predicted by frequency or severity of stuttering. Specifically, through the translation of the Blank Center's distinct **C**ommunication, **A**dvocacy, **R**esiliency, and **E**ducation (**CARE**) framework to clinical practice, participation in Camp DSL empowers children from culturally and linguistically diverse backgrounds who stutter to communicate effectively, speak confidently, and advocate meaningfully so that their daily lives and aspirations are not limited by whether or not they stutter when they speak.

Resilience and Stuttering

Resilience is commonly defined as the ability to recover from setbacks while moving forward with optimism and confidence, or 'the quality of

DOI: 10.4324/9781003179016-5

bouncing back'. Craig et al. (2011) describe it as a "dynamic process in which individuals adjust and cope in an adaptive manner when confronted with significant and threatening adversity (p.1485)." Factors contributing to the development of resilience in children include, among others, internal locus of control, good emotional (self-)regulation, constructive belief patterns (e.g., positive outlook on life), effective coping skills, as well as support networks in one's environment (Benzies & Mychasiuk, 2009). Importantly, some children have a better ability to recover from adverse psycho-social and emotional circumstances, while others need some extra support, but *all* children can become more resilient.

Children with good resilience seek solutions rather than engaging in self-doubt, catastrophic thinking, or victimisation ('Why me?') (Ginsberg & Jablow, 2015). Given that young children who stutter are at risk for the development of negative reactions toward their speech, and may experience negative peer reactions from an early age on (Vanryckeghem et al., 2005), improving resilience is particularly critical in protecting them from developing the higher anxiety, lower self-esteem, lower optimism for the future, and greater victimisation reported by persons who stutter in their later adolescent and adult years (Blood et al., 2011).

Specific intervention programs including a resilience component have been documented to improve the long-term impact of stuttering considerably. Druker et al. (2019) describe how pre-school children whose parents received a resilience component in therapy developed better self-regulation skills, became more resilient themselves, and experienced a reduction in behavioural and emotional problems related to their stuttering. Similar findings have been reported for school-aged children (Caughter & Crofts, 2018), adolescents and adults (Craig et al., 2011).

Negative attitudes toward stuttering and persons who stutter of all ages (Valente et al., 2017) have been documented worldwide. Additionally, Davis et al. (2002) found school-age children who stutter are four times less likely to be considered 'popular' amongst their classmates, two times less likely to be nominated as 'leaders' by their fluent peers, and, at least, three times more likely to experience bullying. The overt behaviour of stuttering is often assumed to be the trigger for the difference in interpersonal relationships, but it is possible that the child who stutters may display an attitude towards his/her speech that yields the peer perception of reduced social status. The more reticent the child feels in social situations, and the less confident they feel in their ability to make friends, puts the child who stutters at greater risk for being an "easy target" for bullying.

As suggested by Byrd et al. (2016), for a child who stutters, the relationship between negative peer evaluation, social anxiety, and bullying can become a 'vicious cycle'. Camp DSL is designed to end this "vicious cycle", by improving children's confidence and competence in their communication, educating them about the nature and development of stuttering, teaching them how to share about stuttering in a way that is empowering and facilitates positive listener perception, and preparing them for challenges they may encounter that are specific to stuttering as well as how to navigate those challenges. The motivating rationale is that if the child who stutters is more competent and confident in their communication, they will be less likely to feel anxious in social settings and more likely to feel positive about their ability to make friends.

Participation in Camp DSL also provides these children with a firm foundation regarding the underlying nature of stuttering, and specific strategies for mitigating the stuttering stereotype. Participants are armed with knowledge of stuttering and how to reduce potential roadblocks that may yield negative thoughts and feelings towards communication both in terms of the listener, as well as in terms of their own perception. Thus, in addition to improving communication, advocacy, and education, participation in Camp DSL builds resilience, and this improvement in the child's ability to navigate the daily and future challenges unique to stuttering is achieved through a variety of unique activities, including improvisation, mindfulness, self-compassion, everyday leaders, paying it forward, peer to peer relationship training.

Improvisation

To prevent stuttering from negatively impacting their everyday life, persons who stutter need to be able to demonstrate stability when they sense they are about to experience a stutter and variability in the manner in which they address that unexpected moment of dysfluency. The use of improvisation training is a key strategy to developing and strengthening resilience (e.g., Rankin et al., 2013). Through improvisation, children who stutter can learn that they cannot anticipate every possible exchange they will have but they can feel comforted by learning that they can respond in a variety of ways, all of which can lead to a successful communicative exchange. Thus, these children will experience positive emotional responses specific to communication which will in turn increase their resilience.

Mindfulness

Given that the relationship between resilience and positive emotional thinking is moderated by negative thoughts (Rosenberg, 2016), Camp DSL also engages the child in group reflection of negative thinking and specifically targets increases in understanding of the value and use of positive self-talk. Researchers have suggested mindfulness training such as Acceptance and Commitment Therapy (e.g., Boyle, 2011; see also Chapter 6) as an effective approach for adults who stutter, but further exploration is needed in children who stutter. Enabling participants in Camp DSL to recognise their thoughts regarding their communication and to learn how to neutralise those thoughts is a critical component to building their resilience.

Self-compassion

In addition to the value of being mindful of negative thinking, studies have also indicated that for children at risk for increased anxiety and low self-confidence, providing opportunities to engage in self-praise that are intended to replace the negative thought patterns they have already developed and/or to counter potential future negative thoughts that could develop over time is of significant benefit to their resilience (Delany et al., 2015). *Camp DSL* addresses expression of these thoughts verbally as well as through art given the research showing that some children are better able to share difficult emotions through artistic outlets (e.g., Gantt & Tinnin, 2009).

Pay It Forward

As is summarised by Byrd and colleagues (e.g., 2016; 2021) another fundamental aspect of *Camp DSL* is the value of helping oneself through helping others. There is a significant body of literature to suggest that the act of helping someone else to cope with the same behaviour with which you have struggled results in increased self-esteem, a deeper connection to the community who would need your help, and also increases self-advocacy (e.g., Anderson & Bigby, 2017). Through helping others, people are more likely to acquire a more profound understanding of their own challenges and how to best navigate similar challenges in the future. Thus, helping others increases resilience.

Camp DSL assigns participants to Pay it Forward peer networks wherein older children who stutter share advice for navigating life as a person who stutters with the younger children in their group. Additionally, on each day of the program participants share what they learned from each other through their interactions in these networks and, together, each network provides specific suggestions for helping other people who stutter whom they have not yet met.

Everyday Leaders

Leadership skills are increased when people are provided with an opportunity to share their life lessons with others who may potentially encounter similar challenges. Leadership skills are also enhanced through the act of teaching others specific skills that the individual has found to be useful (e.g., Martinek & Schilling, 2003). Every child who participates in *Camp DSL* is educated about the importance of leadership. They interact with everyday leaders who review with them what makes a good leader, acknowledge famous leaders, and brainstorm ways to be every day leaders. Each child reflects upon what the everyday leaders share, and they align with the ways in which they lead by example, and the leadership role they envision for themselves in the future.

Research related to the influence of role models on perception of self and future achievement suggest positive effects particularly when the role model has navigated a comparable path whether it be race, gender, intellectual disability, etc. (e.g., Egalite et al., 2015) as the more a person can see success reflected in others who have faced similar challenges, the more positively they will view their own potential. Perhaps of greatest importance, through their interaction with these everyday leaders, they learn that every leader faces challenges, and it is not only how they bounce back from those challenges that defines their success, but also how they perceive themselves as well as how others perceive them – another fundamental component to developing resilience.

Peer to Peer Relationships

Children who experience friendships in preschool and early school age years are less likely to have difficulties with perceptions of self and also less likely to face social isolation (e.g., Laursen et al., 2007). For those children who have not experienced friendships, feelings of insecurity and social inhibition are more likely to develop (e.g., Laird et al., 2001). Through participation in the variety of activities distinct to Camp DSL, children are provided opportunities to bond with each other in meaningful and lasting ways. For example, research has shown that peer relationships in both children and adults are effectively fostered through dance (Brown & Downey, 2009). Dancing facilitates the desire to connect with others (e.g., Deveraux, 2012) and with dancing there is no concern about speech fluency. Thus, dancing is a critical component to Camp DSL.

In addition to dancing, we use art, written expression, small group discussion, and participation in open mic opportunities to establish authentic connections with each other. Across each one of these methods, participants are encouraged to share personal journeys with others with each journey ending with advice for their peers specific to how they can manage the situation if they should ever face the same situation. This process of sharing individual experiences coupled with advice has been documented as a necessary step in the establishment of meaningful bonds. Celebration, laughter and fun is also a fundamental component to the establishment of genuine friendships, therefore, throughout the duration of Camp DSL, children engage in activities designed to ignite joy and humour (Pottie & Sumarah, 2004).

Camp Dream. Speak. Live. Summary

In summary, Camp DSL has been developed to address the affective and cognitive components of stuttering. The treatment protocol includes a variety of distinct opportunities designed to address these components, with activities that independently and collectively improve a child's ability to proactively protect them from and prepare them for adverse experiences unique to stuttering. As is documented in prior studies by Byrd and colleagues, further detailed in Byrd and Hampton (2016), the following targets, general themes and activities comprise the daily schedule for Camp DSL:

1   *Improve communication attitudes and increase resiliency.* Activities designed to improve overall communication attitude are guided by the principle of speaking freely, rather than fluently, across communication exchanges which vary in difficulty. Such activities include open mic events, such as sharing: "What I wish people knew about stuttering" both in front of the camp participants, and in highly trafficked areas. Perseverance and resilience toward self-expression across a variety of environments are also targeted through diverse performance activities, such as a magic show, breakdancing, and improvisation sessions.

2   *Facilitate mentorship and leadership.* To encourage mentorship and leadership, participants are assigned leadership roles, such as leading group activities. Participants are given opportunities to mentor others about stuttering by creating informative and educational messages for parents and peers about stuttering. Activities are designed and varied to offer participants distinct, age-appropriate opportunities for leadership and mentorship.

3   *Improve perception of their ability to establish friendships.* To improve perception of peer relationships, participants engage in complex team problem-solving activities. Open mic activities are designed for reflective peer-to-peer feedback: participants are required to share thoughts and feelings of peers, or to provide feedback on peers' specific talents or traits that make them unique.

4   *Address bullying and teasing.* A motivational speaker and mascot pair are used to promote understanding and navigation of bullying. Participants engage in activities with the speaker mascot pair designed to identify bullying moments, and brainstorm solutions to navigate different teasing situations.

5   *Desensitisation toward stuttering.* To desensitise each child toward stuttering, participants learn about and engage in daily activities such as self-disclosure and voluntary stuttering (see Chapter 7). Additionally, participants are required to reflect upon their speech, completing sentences such as "I love my speech because...."

Participants and parents complete self- and parent-report measures three to seven days before the intervention and again three to fourteen days after the intervention. These measures assess participant communication attitude, participant impact of stuttering on their overall quality of life, and participant and parent perceptions of peer relationships. Behavioural measures include participant performance on core communication competencies. These data are collected on the first and final days of the intervention and analysed post-intervention.

The unique outcomes of Camp DSL have been replicated across multiple studies, suggesting participants' improved communication attitudes and developed more positive perceptions of their ability to form peer-to-peer relationships after participation is statistically and practically significant. Recent findings also demonstrated improved communication competence is achieved, regardless of stuttering frequency. Together, these findings suggest that intensive treatment programs such as Camp DSL – designed specifically to target the psychosocial consequences of childhood stuttering communication skills – positively impact participants' communication attitudes, perceptions of peer relationships, and overall communication effectiveness in a relatively short time frame. Additionally, findings provide additional support to reform treatment guidelines to focus on overall communication competence rather than fluency.

Cross-cultural Case Reports

In the summer of 2014, a young father by the name of Stephen Washington, whose wife was due to have their second child drove from Atlanta, Georgia to Austin, Texas to provide the opportunity for his son, also named Stephen Washington, to attend the initial launch of Camp DSL. Aside from sharing the same bright smiles, Stephen and his son had another similarity - they both stutter. As a father who had experienced stuttering since he was a young child, Stephen was determined to provide his first-born son with opportunities he never had. During his initial inquiry regarding the program, Stephen's overarching goal for his son was that he learns to speak without stuttering, as Stephen felt that was a skill he was never able to attain as a child, despite years of therapy.

Yet, after participating in Camp DSL, rather than speaking fluently, Stephen's son continued to stutter. However, like the published findings have demonstrated, Stephen understood stuttering in a way that put his mind at ease as he felt he was an expert rather than a victim of a circumstance that he was not able to comprehend or explain. He also improved his ability to communicate and advocate, and gained a skill that Stephen's father realised was the most critical skill he was lacking in his own childhood: resilience. Near the end of the weeklong programming, Stephen, age 5, stood up in front of an audience of over 100 people (that included his father) and poignantly shared the following: *"What I learned from my group is, if you stutter, don't give up, just keep on trying and don't let stutters stop you from being who you are."*

Over the last 7 years, both Stephen and his father have continued to stutter, yet, they have accomplished remarkable goals. Stephen tested out of the first grade, travelled to Japan where he learned to speak Japanese fluently, and assumed multiple student and peer leadership roles. His father, through observing the transformation in his son, began to share openly about his own stuttering, and offer lessons regarding communication effectiveness and self-advocacy within his own company where he was recently appointed to an executive leadership position. Together, and individually, they continue to attend Camp DSL but they do so now to help others, as they both want to ensure that stuttering does not stop anyone from being who they are. And, as Stephen, now age 12, shared when he recently served as a peer mentor in our initial launch of Camp DSL in his hometown of Atlanta, Georgia: *"Stuttering can't stop you from living your dreams in your life"*

Although the stigmatisation of stuttering may vary, the pervasive mis-perception that stuttering is something that a person can stop doing, if they try hard enough has been documented worldwide (see Chapter 1). Interestingly, learning about stuttering, enhancing communication skills, and sharing about stuttering in a neutral informative way, have all been shown to yield significant outcomes in persons who stutter from culturally and linguistically diverse populations. Thus, it is not surprising that the positive impact of Camp DSL has been replicated in other countries, such as Ireland, Belgium, and The Netherlands, with several additional countries set to launch in the coming years.

Alice (12 years), a participant in Camp DSL Ireland gave the following feedback: "I have definitely got a lot of positivity and when I go back to school, I will be able to tell the other people that I do stutter and I am ok with it." Fahad (15 years) said that he learned to be confident and that: "you shouldn't be sorry if you stutter, it's just a part of who you are". Thus, like Stephen, and many other children around the world who have participated, Camp DSL facilitated these children to be more resilient, ensuring that they will be able to withstand any ignorance regarding stuttering, so that speaking fluently will never be a prerequisite to them living their lives fully.

Clinicians who participated in the Camp in Ireland work within a free public health system and expressed surprise and satisfaction when following the Camp, many participants and their parents reported that they no longer wished to attend weekly group sessions focused on stuttering modification. These clinicians expressed the view that the increase in communication confidence, along with the acquisition of self-disclosure, resilience, and self-advocacy skills meant that the children no longer focused on trying to fix stuttering but on getting on with their lives. This has implications for of-fering more effective therapy as opposed to higher doses of therapy focused on changing stuttering behaviours.

Conclusion

Most children who stutter who are still stuttering at age 7 will likely persist in their stuttering, whether they receive treatment or not. Chronic stuttering can lead to significant negative academic, emotional, social, and vocational out-comes as an adult. However, these outcomes are not the result of experiences in adulthood, rather many adults report that they began in their early child-hood through experiencing bullying and diminished peer relationships, and experiences that substantially affected their lives decades later. Thus, treatment approaches for children who stutter should address the affective and cognitive consequences of persistent stuttering early in life, to proactively prevent or, at least, better equip them for and/or reduce challenges later in life.

Camp DSL bolsters children's communication skills, and positively impacts their communication attitudes, and their understanding of stuttering. Attendance provides them with empowering strategies for sharing about stuttering with others, as well as improving their perceptions of their ability to meaningfully establish peer relationships, all of which strengthens their resilience, or rather their capacity for navigating the adversity they may face specific to their stuttering. In sum, every participant is taught that what they have to say is important, and to never let stuttering stop them from pursuing their dreams, speaking from their hearts, and living their life to the fullest. Hence, the intensive program name, "Camp Dream. Speak. Live."

References

Anderson, S. & Bigby, C. (2017). Self-advocacy as a means to positive identities for people with intellectual disability: 'We just help them, be them really'. *Journal of Applied Research in Intellectual Disabilities*. 30 (1), 109–120. 10.1111/jar.12223

Benzies, K. & Mychasiuk, R. (2009). Fostering family resiliency: a review of the key protective factors. *Child and Family Social Work*. 14, 103–114. 10.1111/j.1365-2206.2 008.00586.x

Blood, G. W., Blood, I. M., Tramontana, G. M., Sylvia, A. J., Boyle, M. P., & Motzko, G. R. (2011). Self-reported experience of bullying of students who stutter: Relations with life satisfaction, life orientation, and self-esteem. *Perceptual and Motor Skills*. 113 (2), 353–364.

Boyle M. P. (2011). Mindfulness training in stuttering therapy: a tutorial for speech-language pathologists. *Journal of fluency disorders*. 36 (2), 122–129. 10.1016/j.jfludis. 2011.04.005

Brown, C. & Downey, L., (2009). From the 2008 Research Poster Session at the American Dance Therapy Association 43rd Annual Conference. *American Journal of Dance Therapy*. 31 (1), 64–70.

Byrd, C. T., Hampton, E., McGill, M., & Gkalitsiou, Z. (2016). Participation in Camp Dream. Speak. Live: Affective and Cognitive Outcomes for Children who Stutter. *Journal of Speech Pathology and Therapy*. 1, 116. 10.4172/2472-5005.1000116

Byrd, C. T. & Hampton, E. (2016). *Camp Dream. Speak. Live.: An Intensive Therapy Program for Children Who Stutter*. Austin, TX: UT Copy Services.

Byrd C. T.,Gkalitsiou, Z., Werle, D., & Coalson, G. A. (2018). Exploring the effectiveness of an intensive treatment program for school-age children who stutter, Camp Dream. Speak. Live.: a follow-up study. *Seminars in Speech and Language*. 39 (05), 458–468.

Byrd, C. T., Winters, K. L., Young, M., Werle, D., Croft, R. L., Hampton, E., Coalson, G.A., White, A., & Gkalitsiou, Z. (2021). The Communication Benefits of Participation in Camp Dream. Speak. Live.: An Extension and Replication. *Seminars in Speech and Language*. 42(02), 117–135. 10.1055/s-0041-1723843

Caughter, S. & Crofts, V. (2018). Nurturing a resilient mindset in school-aged children who stutter. American *Journal of Speech-Language Pathology*. 27 (3S), 1111–1123. 10.1044/2018_AJSLP-ODC11-17-0189

Craig, A., Blumgart, E., & Tran, Y. (2011). Resilience and stuttering: Factors that protect people from the adversity of chronic stuttering. *Journal of Speech Language and Hearing Research*. 54 (6), 1485–1496. 10.1044/1092-4388(2011/10-0304)

Davis, S., Howell, P., & Cooke, F. (2002). Sociodynamic relationships between children who stutter and their non-stuttering classmates. *Journal of Child Psychology and Psychiatry*. 43 (7), 939–947. 10.1111/1469-7610.00093

Delany, C., Miller, K. J., El-Ansary, D., Remedios, L., Hosseini, A., & McCleod, S. (2015). Replacing stressful challenges with positive coping strategies: A resilience program for clinical placement learning. *Advances in Health Sciences Education: Theory and Practice*. 20, 1301–1324. 10.1007/s10459-015-9603-3

Deveraux, C. (2012). Moving Into Relationships: Dance/Movement Therapy With Children With Autism. In *Play-based interventions for children and adolescents with autism spectrum disorders* (pp. 361–380). Routledge.

Druker, K. C., Mazzuchelli, T. G., & Beilby, J. M. (2019). An evaluation of an integrated fluency and resilience program for early developmental stuttering disorders. *Journal of Communication Disorders*. 78, 69–83.

Egalite, A. J., Kisida, B., & Winters, M. A. (2015). Representation in the classroom: The effect of own-race teachers on student achievement. *Economics of Education Review*. 45, 44–52.

Gantt, L. & Tinnin, L. W. (2009). Support for a neurobiological view of trauma with implications for art therapy. *The Arts in Psychotherapy*. 36 (3), 148–153. 10.1016/j.aip. 2008.12.005

Ginsberg, K. R. & Jablow, M. M. (2015). *Building resilience in children and teens: Giving kids roots and wings* (3rd Ed.). Elk Grove Village (IL): American Academy of Pediatrics.

Laird, R. D., Jordan, K. Y., Dodge, K. A., Pettit, G. S., & Bates, J. E. (2001). Peer rejection in childhood, involvement with antisocial peers in early adolescence, and the development of externalizing behavior problems. *Development and psychopathology*. 13 (2), 337–354. 10.1017/s0954579401002

Laursen, B., Bukowski, W. M., Aunola, K., & Nurmi, J. E. (2007). Friendship moderates prospective associations between social isolation and adjustment problems in young children. *Child development*. 78 (4), 1395–1404. 10.1111/j.1467-8624.2007.01072.x

Martinek, T. & Schilling, T. (2003). Developing compassionate leadership in underserved youths. *Journal of Physical Education, Recreation & Dance*. 74 (5), 33–39. 10.1080/07303084. 2003.1060848

O'Dwyer, M., Walsh, I. P., & Leahy, M. M. (2018). The Role of Narratives in the Development of Stuttering as a Problem. *American Journal of Speech and Language Pathology*. 27 (3S), 1164–1179. 10.1044/2018_AJSLP-ODC11-17-0207

Pottie, C. & Sumarah, J. (2004). Friendships between persons with and without developmental disabilities. *Mental retardation*. 42(1), 55–66. 10.1352/0047-6765(2004)42<55: FBPWAW>2.0.CO;2

Rankin, A., Dahlbäck, N., & Lundberg, J., (2013). A case study of factor influencing role improvisation in crisis response teams. *Cognition, technology & work*. 15 (1), 79–93. 10.1007/s10111-011-0186-3

Rosenberg, A. (2016). Foster resilience in adolescent and young adult cancer patients. *Oncology Times*. 38, 8–9.

Valente, A., St Louis, K. O., Leahy, M., Hall, A., & Jesus, L. (2017). A country-wide probability sample of public attitudes toward stuttering in Portugal. *Journal of fluency disorders.* 52, 37–52. 10.1016/j.jfludis.2017.03.001

Vanryckeghem, M., Brutten, G. J., & Hernandez, L. M. (2005). A comparative investigation of the speech-associated attitude of preschool and kindergarten children who do and do not stutter. *Journal of Fluency Disorders.* 30, 307–318.

6 Cognitive Approaches with Children who Stutter and their Parents

Elaine Kelman, Ali Berquez, and Sarah Caughter

Introduction

Cognitive approaches have long been used to support clients who stutter, typically within a holistic therapeutic model. Here, we outline the development of cognitive therapy over time, discuss the use of third generation approaches including Acceptance and Commitment Therapy (ACT, Hayes, 2004; Webster, 2018), Mindfulness (Kabat-Zinn, 1996), and Compassion Focused Therapy (CFT, Gilbert, 2009; 2010; Neff, 2003b), within the context of the Palin Model, 2019 (www.michaelpalincentreforstammering.org), and consider practical applications with children and young people who stutter, and their parents.

First generation CBT was used in the 1940s as a short-term treatment for depression and anxiety, based on principles of classical conditioning and operant learning, along with the theory that cognitions lead to dysfunctional behaviours; so, altering cognitions can lead to positive behaviour change. Cognitive Behaviour Therapy (CBT, 'second generation') was developed in the 1960s (Beck, 1967) for clients with depression. Beckian CBT has a robust evidence-base with adults (Hofmann et al., 2012) and application with children and young people has evolved over the past 15–20 years for a range of mental health difficulties (Kelman & Wheeler, 2015).

Key aspects of early CBT included identifying a client's negative automatic thoughts (NATs) and emotional responses and the relationship they had in influencing physiological responses and behaviour (a vicious cycle). Each psychological disorder is described by a disorder-specific model to facilitate understanding of salient maintenance factors, with a particular emphasis on thoughts as the driver for behavioural responses. Therapy includes identifying NATs; recognising unhelpful thinking patterns; testing or challenging NATs or thinking of more helpful and adaptive ways of viewing negative thinking, and use of behavioural experiments.

Third generation approaches have shifted the focus away from challenging negative thinking patterns towards developing a different relationship with these uncomfortable thoughts and feelings and building psychological flexibility. This has led to clients moving away from suppression, avoidance,

DOI: 10.4324/9781003179016-6

thought testing and challenge; towards developing mindful attention, curiosity, kindness and acceptance about their thoughts, beliefs, feelings and behaviours, thus enabling clients to live life in a way that is personally meaningful to them (Hayes, 2004). This shift has brought a novel opportunity for clients to consider their stuttering in a different way (Boyle, 2011; Beilby et al., 2012; Harley, 2015, 2018; Cheasman et al., 2015). Instead of trying to avoid feelings of anxiety or trying to suppress worries about the cost of stuttering and how others might perceive or judge them, clients are encouraged to notice their thoughts and feelings, to sit with them, to become curious about them and to develop distance from them. Mindfulness develops the practice of being aware of the present moment, noticing and sitting with difficult thoughts and emotions, whilst nurturing a mindset of kindness and curiosity. This elegantly complements Gilbert's work in CFT, in supporting clients who experience shame and self-criticism, to practise self-warmth and inner compassion.

Third generation approaches have supported clients to use language that validates and normalises their experiences and emotions. Within an ACT framework, the language used is non-judgmental, compassionate and accepting; for instance, 'noticing' thoughts rather than *changing them;* describing thoughts in a kinder and more curious way (e.g., 'what your brain is saying to you') rather than as *dysfunctional, irrational* or *faulty.* ACT and mindfulness fit well within the social model of disability discourse, enabling each person to determine what is personally meaningful to them (Bailey et al., 2015). Shifting the relationship with thoughts and feelings is a welcome development in stuttering therapy and has been shown to enhance psychological well-being, with positive gains maintained over time (Beilby et al., 2012).

Theoretical Context

In 2019 the Michael Palin Centre team developed the Palin Model as a framework for understanding stuttering and its assessment and therapy. The core of the Palin Model (Figure 6.1) is an image of the child or young person with his brain as the focal point of why he stutters. This represents the physiological factors, including genetic and neurological factors as the underlying explanation for stuttering. Stuttering may also be influenced by physical factors such as motor coordination or physical wellbeing, including health and tiredness. The child is within a triangle and at each point are influencing factors: speech motor; language and communication; and psychological. These represent the child's skills and vulnerabilities, which may influence the development and impact of stuttering. The outer circle represents the child's home, school or social environment. Environmental influences interact with the other factors to compound or diminish stuttering. The Palin Model provides a framework for assessment of the child's strengths and vulnerabilities and what may be influencing stuttering, which then informs the individualised therapy plan. The Palin Model is shared with the child and parents to facilitate an open, collaborative therapeutic relationship with the family.

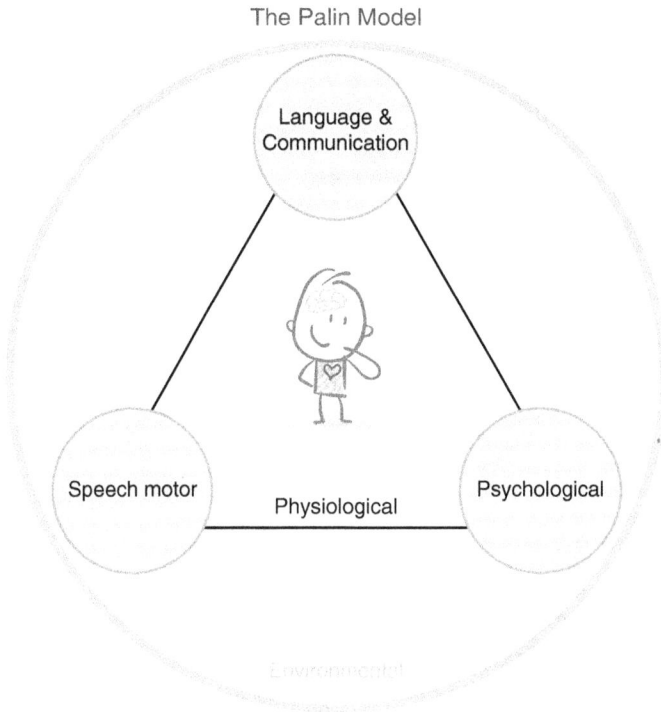

Figure 6.1 The Palin model.

The child's psychological profile is an integral component of our under-standing of stuttering and comprises the child's temperament, the cognitive and affective impact of stuttering and how these interact with aspects of the child's functioning and their environment. This will consequently shape the nature of therapy and what is included. The psychological components of therapy are interwoven and involve the child's system. Over the years these have been heavily influenced by CBT (Beck, 1967), Solution Focused Brief Therapy (de Shazer, 1985, 1996; Ratner et al., 2012) and more recently 'third generation' approaches including ACT (Webster, 2018), Mindfulness (Kabat-Zinn, 1996) and CFT (Gilbert, 2009; 2010; Neff, 2003b).

The Social Disability Model as it relates to stuttering (Bailey et al., 2015), differentiates between a person's impairment (in this case, stuttering) and the disability that a person with an impairment experiences due to the physical, structural and cultural barriers they face. These barriers include societal stereotypes and negative attitudes, as well as beliefs held by the person who stutters - the self-stigma, reinforced by external values (Boyle, 2013). Stuttering is viewed as a different way of communicating, rather than being 'dysfunctional'; and 'neurodiversity' is used to describe the neurological differences that underlie stuttering.

The Social Disability Model has challenged us to achieve a balance between helping children, young people and their parents to feel that stuttering is acceptable and does not define an individual nor limit their possibilities (Campbell et al., 2019), whilst offering support towards acceptance, increased agency, confidence and resilience (Caughter & Crofts, 2018), greater ease and enjoyment of communication and improved participation in life. Speech fluency is not a requirement for successful communication; thus, therapy addresses the cognitive and affective components of stuttering, openness and desensitisation. It also includes developing the child's social communication skills and increasing their comfort and ease of talking when stuttering. Furthermore, clinicians have an important role in challenging the stereotypes held by society - within families, schools and across the media.

Cognitive Approaches in Practice

Establishing a Direction of Travel

A key aspect of any therapeutic intervention is to establish what a client wants from therapy. ACT helps clients to make choices about what they want (the choice point) and where they want to be, in line with their values ('towards moves'); and to recognise what is not working for them and may be taking them in an undesired direction ('away moves') (Polk et al., 2016). This process puts the client at the centre of clinical decision making. As described by Hayes (2004, p. 19), *"the therapeutic relationship is important, powerful, and deliberately equal in ACT"*.

Many children and young people who stutter, and their parents, tell us they want to stop stuttering. We aim to support each client to reach their potential, whether they continue to stutter or not. A challenge is to balance the tension between meeting a client's hopes without fostering unrealistic expectations. Warren, a 9-year-old who stutters, tells us he wants to "get rid of" his stuttering. He tells us he wants to talk like his peers, to take part in conversations, tell jokes and have a technique to manage his stutter. We support him to 'lean in' to moments of stuttering so that he sits with it rather than tries to avoid it, to become desensitised to it, to explore the advantages and disadvantages of techniques, and to reduce the struggle and tension he experiences during moments of stuttering. It is important that we respect what he wants from therapy, individualise his therapy and go at his pace.

ACT is a behavioural approach and therefore an important aspect of therapy is behaviour change e.g., doing more of what is important to you. For children and young people who stutter this may be talking more in class, interacting more with friends, or ordering the food they want to eat, rather than what's easiest to say. These ideas can be explored throughout therapy and celebrated when clients notice 'towards moves' in line with their values.

Paying Attention to Thoughts and Feelings

Mindfulness is widely used and integrated into work with children and young people (e.g., the Mindfulness in Schools Project, MiSP, in the UK for 3–18-year-olds, https://mindfulnessinschools.org). Mindful breathing helps clients to focus on the breath, to slow down and to learn to be more present. For clients who stutter, mindfulness encourages them to notice and sit with their discomfort rather than escape or suppress it.

Exercises for children such as 'Breathing Buddies' and 'Finger Breathing' are highly visual and can therefore support younger children. One 6-year-old client who stutters, Emily, was invited to find a favourite toy (her polar bear) and place it on her stomach so she could notice the rise and fall of her stomach when breathing (Breathing Buddy) and to enjoy this experience with her 'buddy' as a helper. Her mother practised mindfulness exercises with her using the resource *Sitting Still Like a Frog* (Snel, 2013) in order to develop a daily mindful practice. A group of ten- to 14-year-olds who stutter were taught to trace the slow inhalation and exhalation of the breath using their fingers (Finger Breathing). As they breathed in they traced upwards along each finger, at their own pace, and as they exhaled they traced downwards on each finger. The outbreath enabled them to notice the release of tension.

Bibliotherapy has been recognised as a powerful adjunct to therapy, facilitating carry-over of skills into everyday life. Children who stutter are helped by understanding that worry is common to most people and that people who don't stutter also experience anxiety. Use of stories such as *Ruby's Worry* (Percival, 2018) and *Worrysaurus* (Bright & Chatterton, 2019) are a child-friendly, and visual way, of exploring thoughts and feelings, and by re-enacting or re-writing the story, drawing or painting it, and thinking about the take-home messages of the story, clients can consider how this might apply to their own experience (Pearson & Kordich Hall, 2006).

Sitting with Thoughts and Feelings

ACT and mindfulness approaches encourage clients who stutter to sit alongside, 'unhook', or disentangle themselves, from difficult and habitual thoughts and to practise being present. The concept of *cognitive defusion* promotes distancing from thoughts. This is a useful practice for clients who stutter as it enables them to 'lean in' to the experience of stuttering, to be aware of the tendency towards avoidance or suppression, and ensuing struggle, and to sit with this tension. Snow globes or glitter jars are helpful visual resources to use with children, to understand the experience of anxiety that can be exacerbated by stuttering. Watching a snow globe or glitter jar when shaken, gives the clinician the opportunity to discuss how anxiety tends to increase rapidly then gradually reduces over time (as the snow or glitter settles). This is powerfully illustrated in 'Just Breathe' (Salzman & Salzman, 2014). The analogy of a closed door (that we want to push through) or bubble wrap (that we want to pop) can help to discuss how tempting it is to push and how hard it can be to resist.

Allowing thoughts to come and go, and being curious about them from a distance, can be empowering. Yusuf, a 14-year-old client, found the analogy of watching his thoughts float by, as if on clouds, a helpful visualisation. He described how some could be dark and angry, and others lighter and softer, but he watched them all floating by. Psychological distancing from thoughts enables us to see thoughts as 'just thoughts' and reduces their negative impact.

By making therapy activities fun, practical and concrete we are more likely to engage younger clients. Warren, aged 9, was asked to recall what it felt like when he tried to hold a beach ball underwater. He described the tension in his muscles, the effort involved and the explosion in an unpredictable direction when he let it go, or it escaped his grasp. He then discussed what it was like when the beach ball rested on the water's surface being blown gently by the wind as a way to explore advantages of leaning into the experience of stuttering instead of trying to hide it or push through it.

A group of 10- to 14-year-old children, and their parents, were encouraged to think of a worry and place it on their hand, put their hand up close to their face, then gradually move their hand further away. This acts as a visual representation of distancing. Similarly, when they notice a worry, they create distance from it by saying to themselves: 'my mind is telling me that…'". Another cognitive defusion exercise involves repeating a word over and over again until the meaning becomes lost, and distance is established from the literal meaning (e.g., the 'Milk Exercise', Hayes & Wilson, 1994). A 15-year-old client, Tom, found this particularly helpful when practising saying his name: viewing it as a series of sounds that he was able to say, thus distancing himself from uncomfortable memories of repeatedly blocking on his name. The analogy of the 'passengers on a bus' is another helpful way of recognising how our thoughts and emotions (the passengers) can hijack the direction we travel in. This was used with a 19-year-old, Georgie, who reflected that "not engaging with the rowdy passengers" (the negative thoughts) on her bus had helped her to speak her mind when it mattered to her ('a towards move').

Desensitisation

The process of becoming more attuned to thoughts and feelings and shifting the relationship with them facilitates a process of desensitisation towards the experience of stuttering. It enables clients to experiment with being more open, and for parents to acknowledge and talk about stuttering (Berquez & Kelman, 2018), to become more knowledgeable about stuttering, to consider that it's okay to stutter, to discuss differences and to develop self-advocacy.

We talk to our clients about value-laden language and how that impacts on the client's, and others', perceptions (Kelman & Nicholas, 2020). This can send a powerful message to the client themselves, and also to their family and friends, that it is ok to stutter. It is often helpful to agree what to call stuttering. Whilst a pre-school child might talk about 'sticky' or 'bumpy' sounds and words, we find it helpful to call stuttering what it is, even with young children, and to discuss this as one difference, alongside many others. We explore how each person has differences, to give the message that each person is unique, we are all different and we all have strengths and vulnerabilities. Emily, aged six, and her mother generated a list of differences about people. They also read and discussed the story of *Giraffes Can't Dance* (Andreae & Parker-Rees, 2000) which has the helpful message: 'sometimes when we're different we just need a different song'. Emily concluded that we are all different and unique, like our fingerprints, and her toy unicorn.

As we discuss terminology about stuttering, that it is ok to talk about it and acknowledge it and that we all have differences, we equip each child to explain stuttering to peers. At the start of therapy with Mimi, aged 6, she wanted to tell her peers she saw a doctor each week and her parents wanted to take her back to school in breaktime so no one would ask where she had been, enabling a conspiracy of silence (Gould & Sheehan, 1967). She was supported to advocate for herself, to tell peers she stutters, to describe stuttering and to explain what helped. She explained to her peers "I see someone to help me with my stutter, when my words get stuck...it helps when you listen and wait". She concluded this helped her classmates to understand her more. Emily, aged six, explained to her parents that stuttering "happens in my brain, on the left-hand side, and though I want to talk fast I have to talk slow"; and then explained to her brother: "just because I speak a bit differently doesn't mean I'm not normal".

Amplifying the Kinder Voice

Compassion Focused Therapy (CFT, Gilbert, 2009, 2010; Neff, 2003b) promotes self-compassion and kindness. Useful questions include 'What would you say to a friend?' to enable third person perspective-taking and to promote helpful self-talk. Self-compassion can be developed from a young age. Normalising mistakes and viewing them as an opportunity for growth and learning helps children to be kinder to themselves. *Your Fantastic Elastic Brain* (Deak & Ackerley, 2010) develops understanding about the complexities of talking, our 'amazing' brains, and how they develop. After reading this book Emily, six, commented: "mistakes help our brain grow", and "your brain stretches like an elastic band when you're being brave". *Beautiful Oops!* (Saltzberg, 2010) reframes mistakes as possibilities and can be helpful in cognitive reframing; and *The Dot* (Reynolds, 2003), where a child thinks she can't draw then discovers she can, are useful tools to facilitate discussion with younger children.

The 'Coach' analogy (Hoffman & Otto, 2008) can support more balanced and positive perspective taking. Nathan, an 18-year-old who stutters, became highly preoccupied by post-event rumination about stuttering and expressed concern about listener judgement. He found the concept of 'Coach A' (the harshly critical voice) versus 'Coach B' (the kinder voice) helpful in reflecting which 'coach' is likely to allow us to perform at our best which enabled him to generate a kinder message to himself. He concluded that "we can't know how the listener may have been thinking" and "they seemed to enjoy the conversation". He reflected that thinking about what 'Coach B' might say helped him to reflect on the experience with greater self-compassion, which ultimately enabled a positive shift in his mood and behaviour.

Conclusion

Similarities and differences exist in the cognitive approaches discussed here and whilst ACT and CBT have different theoretical underpinnings, they may be used in a complementary or 'hybrid' way (Harley, 2015) to enrich the therapeutic experience of children and young people who stutter. These psychological approaches enable clinicians to offer a flexible and holistic approach and support clients to explore and experiment with noticing unhelpful thinking, tolerating difficult emotions, sitting with uncomfortable thoughts and practising psychological distancing from them. The activities described in this chapter are examples from clients who are attending therapy at the Centre and should be considered within the wider context of the ACT theoretical framework and within a holistic therapy approach with children and their families, as outlined in the Palin Model.

The range of cognitive approaches, from Beckian CBT which changes unhelpful thinking to ACT which makes room for negative thoughts and feelings, provides many options for therapy with children and young people who stutter and their families. We must ensure that therapy is engaging, tailored to the child's individual needs and interests and has a practical and experiential focus. If our clients (and their parents) are able to relate to their thoughts about stuttering differently, and more compassionately, they may be better equipped to reach their full potential.

References

Andreae, G. & Parker-Rees, G. (2000). *Giraffes Can't Dance*. Orchard Books.

Bailey, K., Harris, S. J., & Simpson, S. (2015). Stammering and the social model of disability: Challenge and opportunity. *Procedia—Social and Behavioral Sciences*. 193, 13–24. 10.1016/j.sbspro.2015.03.240

Beck, A. T. (1967). *Depression: Causes and treatment*. Philadelphia: University of Pennsylvania Press.

Berquez, A. & Kelman, E. (2018). Methods in Stuttering Therapy for Desensitising Parents of Children who Stutter. *American Journal of Speech and Language Pathology*. 27, p1124–p1138. 10.1044/2018_AJSLP-ODC11-17-0183

Beilby, J. M., Byrnes, M. L., & Yaruss, S. (2012). Acceptance and Commitment Therapy for adults who stutter: psychosocial adjustment and speech fluency, *Journal of Fluency Disorders*. 37 (4), 289–299. 10.1016/j.jfludis.2012.05.003

Boyle, M. P. (2011). Mindfulness training in stuttering therapy: A tutorial for speech-language pathologists. *Journal of Fluency Disorders*. 36 (2), 122–129. 10.1016/j.jfludis. 2011.04.005

Boyle M. P. (2013). Assessment of stigma associated with stuttering: development and evaluation of the self-stigma of stuttering scale (4S). *Journal of Speech Language Hearing Research, Oct.* 56 (5), 1517–1529. 10.1044/1092-4388(2013/12-0280)

Bright. R. & Chatterton, C. (2019). *Worrysaurus*. UK: Orchard Books.

Campbell, P., Constantino, C., & Simpson, S. (2019). *Stammering Pride and Prejudice. Difference not Defect.* J&R Press.

Caughter, S. & Crofts, V. (2018) Nurturing a resilient mindset in school-aged children who stutter. *American Journal of Speech and Language Pathology*. 27, 1111–1123. 10.1044/2018_AJSLP-ODC11-17-0189

Cheasman, C., Simpson, S., & Everard, R. (2015). Acceptance and speech work: the challenge. *Procedia - Social and Behavioral Sciences*. 193 (2015), 72– 81. 10.1016/j.sbspro. 2015.03.246

Deak, J. & Ackerley, S. (2010). *Your Fantastic Elastic Brain: Stretch It, Shape It*. Little Pickle Press.

de Shazer, S. (1985). *Keys to Solutions in Brief Therapy*. W. W. Norton & Company

de Shazer, S. (1996). *Words Were Originally Magic*. Norton, New York.

Gilbert, P. (2010). *The compassionate mind: A new approach to life's challenges*. New Harbinger Publications.

Gilbert, P. (2009). Introducing compassion-focused therapy. *Advances in Psychiatric Treatment*. 15 (3), 199–208. 10.1192/apt.bp.107.005264

Gould, E. & Sheehan, O. (1967). Effect of silence on stuttering, *Journal of Abnormal Psychology*. 72, 441–445. 10.1037/h0025088

Harley, J. (2018). The role of attention in therapy for children and adolescents who stutter: cognitive-behaviour therapy and mindfulness-based interventions. *American Journal of Speech and Language Pathology*. 27, 1139–1151. 10.1044/2018_AJSLP-ODC11-17-0196

Harley, J (2015). Bridging the Gap between Cognitive Therapy and Acceptance and Commitment Therapy (ACT). Proceedings of the 10th Oxford Dysfluency Conference 17–20 July 2014. *Procedia Social and Behavioral Sciences*, pp. 13–140. 10.1016/j.sbspro. 2015.03.252

Hayes, S. C. & Wilson, K. G. (1994). Acceptance and Commitment Therapy: Altering the Verbal Support for Experiential Avoidance. *The Behaviour Analyst*. 17, 289–303. 10.1007/BF03392677

Hayes, S. C. (2004). Acceptance and Commitment Therapy, Relational Frame Theory, and the third wave of behavioral and cognitive therapies. *Behavior Therapy*. 35, 639–665. 10.1016/S0005-7894(04)80013-3

Hoffman, S. G. & Otto, M. W. (2008). *Cognitive Behavioral Therapy for Social Anxiety Disorder: Evidence-based and Disorder-specific Treatment Techniques*. New York, NY: Routledge.

Hofmann, S. G., Asnaani, A., Vonk, I. J., Sawyer, A. T., & Fang, A. (2012). The Efficacy of Cognitive Behavioral Therapy: A Review of Meta-analyses. *Cognitive therapy and research*. 36 (5), 427–440. 10.1007/s10608-012-9476-1

Kabat-Zinn, J. (1996). *Full catastrophe living*. London: Piatkus.

Kelman, E. & Nicholas, A. (2020). *Palin Parent-Child Interaction Therapy for Early Stammering*. Speechmark.

Kelman, E. & Wheeler, S. (2015). Cognitive Behaviour Therapy with Children. *Procedia - Social and Behavioral Sciences*. 195, 165–174. 10.1016/j.sbspro.2015.03.256

Mindfulness in Schools Project: https://mindfulnessinschools.org

Neff, K. D. (2003b). Self-compassion: An alternative conceptualization of a healthy attitude toward oneself. *Self and Identity*. 2, 85–102. 10.1080/15298860309032

Palin Model (2019). www.michaelpalincentreforstammering.org

Pearson, J. & Kordich Hall, D. (2006). *Reaching In...Reaching Out: Resiliency Guidebook*. http://www.reachinginreachingout.com/resources-guidebook.htm

Percival, T. (2018). *Ruby's Worry: A big bright feelings book*. Bloomsbury.

Polk, K. L. Schoendorff, B., Webster, M., & Olaz, F. O. (2016). *The Essential Guide to the ACT Matrix: A Step-by-Step Approach to Using the ACT Matrix Model in Clinical Practice*. United Kingdom: New Harbinger Publications.

Ratner, H., George, E., & Iveson, C. (2012). *Solution focused brief therapy: 100 key points and techniques*. Routledge.

Reynolds, P. H. (2003). *The Dot*. Candlewick Press

Saltzberg, B. (2010). *Beautiful Oops!*. New York: Workman Publishing.

Salzman, J. B. & Salzman, J. (2014). *Just Breathe* https://www.youtube.com/watch?v=-YEZnrySrtQ

Snel, E. (2013). *Sitting Still Like a Frog: Mindfulness Exercises for Kids (and their Parents)* with CD ROM. Shambhala Publications Inc.

Webster, M. (2018). Introduction to acceptance and commitment therapy. *Advances in Psychiatric Treatment*. 17 (4), July 2011, 309– 316. 10.1192/apt.bp.107.005256

7 Working with Adults Who Stutter

Michael Blomgren

Introduction

Stuttering is a multidimensional disorder (Bennett, 2006; Smith & Kelly, 1997). This multidimensionality indicates that stuttering is a complex disorder, belying simple explanations as to aetiology and treatment. Stuttering is thought to arise from a combination of genetic, neurological and developmental influences. The neurological components explain aspects of the chronic nature of the disorder in adolescents and adults.

The auditory and visually observable core elements of stuttering include the speech motor behaviours of repeated articulatory movements (e.g., t-t-t-talk) and fixed articulatory postures (e.g., mmmine) (Teesson et al., 2003). In addition, stuttering moments are often accompanied by muscle tension and other secondary, nonverbal gestures such as facial grimaces, eye blinking and loss of eye contact. While the core and secondary features of stuttering are those most readily visible to an observer, stuttering is more than its surface manifestations. Aspects of stuttering that are not as immediately evident include affective and emotional aspects of stuttering (Blomgren, 2007).

Although stuttering may have biological origins, factors such as anxiety may influence the severity and the variability of the disorder. Approximately 50% of adults who stutter may have significantly high levels of social anxiety (Kraaimaat et al., 2002; Menzies et al., 2008). Stuttering speakers often develop numerous avoidance strategies such as avoiding 'difficult' words, avoiding stressful speaking situations, or avoiding talking with people where a history of excessive stuttering exists. For many who stutter, avoidance behaviours may hinder social and occupational participation and increase anxiety, feelings of frustration, embarrassment, self-doubt and shame related to stuttering (Blumgart et al., 2010; Gabel et al., 2008).

The goals of stuttering treatment should address the physical tension related to speaking and the challenges to social participation and mental well-being. Specifically, a comprehensive approach to treating stuttering includes addressing core stuttering behaviours, secondary behaviours and possible anxiety and avoidance-related consequences of stuttering.

DOI: 10.4324/9781003179016-7

Stuttering Therapy

The first step in providing appropriate and relevant treatment is conducting a robust assessment of the client's stuttering pattern, assessing the personal and vocational consequences of the stuttering, and determining the client's goals for treatment. Stuttering assessment includes interviewing a client to understand why they are seeking help so that you can collaboratively create an effective individualised treatment plan.

While numerous therapy approaches exist to help people who stutter, many can be separated into two broad categories: (1) 'stuttering management' (also known as 'stuttering modification') and (2) 'speech restructuring' (also known as 'fluency shaping'). Stuttering management therapies focus, besides the modification of stuttering moments, on the cognitive, emotional, social, vocational and avoidance issues related to stuttering. In contrast, speech restructuring therapies focus primarily on teaching a new speech motor pattern that facilitates fluent speech (Blomgren, 2010). Speech restructuring therapy has the most robust empirical evidence base. The evidence base for stuttering management approaches tends to be inferred from work in cognitive behaviour therapy and desensitisation. Comprehensive approaches for treating stuttering in adults address both improved speech fluency and stuttering management.

There is disagreement regarding the essential components of stuttering treatment for adults (Blomgren et al., 2005; Blomgren et al., 2006b; Blomgren et al., 2006a; Reitzes & Snyder, 2006; Ryan, 2006). However, the long-term popularity of many of these diverse treatment approaches may indicate their varied benefits for different groups of people who stutter. For example, decreasing anxiety related to stuttering is the primary concern for some people who stutter, while others primarily want to speak more fluently.

Many factors may play a role in determining the best course of therapy. One issue is the time available to the client. Some therapy approaches, such as speech restructuring, may necessitate many treatment hours and long-term dedication to practice. For instance, some intensive speech restructuring programs involve 50–100 hours of learning speech techniques and related training. For many clients, the costs of these programs are prohibitive in terms of time and money. In general, when treatment hours are limited, it may be most practical to focus on stuttering management approaches or simplified speech restructuring techniques. As the availability of treatment time increases, the attention to speech restructuring can likewise increase.

Stuttering Management

Stuttering management therapies encompass a broad range of techniques, including anxiety reduction and modification of stuttering moments. The end goal of many of these techniques is desensitisation to stuttering. Other strategies focus on stuttering modification techniques designed to reduce muscular tension associated with stuttering moments. Stuttering management therapies started in the 1930s with Lee Travis and Bryng Bryngelson and were re-searched, refined and popularised by Van Riper (1973). This treatment required attitude change and social adjustment to help the client deal with the social and vocational consequences of stuttering. Like most desensitisation therapies, stuttering management therapy has its origin in the cognitive learning literature. The main goals of stuttering management therapy are to develop acceptance of stuttering, reduce fear and anxiety associated with stuttering and to teach the person who stutters to stutter with decreased effort (Blomgren, 2012).

Disclosure of Stuttering

Disclosure of one's stuttering is an essential stuttering management technique (Lee & Manning, 2010; Healey et al., 2007). Disclosing stuttering is simply advertising the fact that one is not a fluent speaker. Many people who stutter spend much of their speaking time trying to hide their stuttering, and this constant process of hiding and avoidance can be stressful and tiring. People who stutter may try to hide their stuttering out of embarrassment, poor acceptance of their disorder, or perhaps even out of simple habit. Regardless of the reason, actively hiding a stutter is counterproductive to stress-free communication.

There are two primary goals in having a client openly disclose their stutter. First, by letting a listener know what is occurring, a stuttering speaker will be displaying that they are comfortable and confident despite their disorder. Second, when a listener knows what is going on – that the behaviour they are observing is stuttering – they will be less likely to be uncomfortable and embarrassed.

Disclosure takes practice and dedication. It is helpful to role-play different ways to disclose stuttering with a client. Clients will only use an approach that is comfortable for them. Breitenfeldt and Lorenz (1999) described three methods to disclosure. The first, and perhaps the easiest, is the direct route, where a client states something like, "my name is Michael and I stutter." The script must feel socially appropriate for the client. Another method is using humour to lighten the mood. Seeing the humour in stuttering can be challenging for many, but being able to laugh at a moment of stuttering can also be a powerful act of desensitisation. The final approach is voluntary stuttering. This technique involves stuttering on purpose in a controlled way. This pseudo-stuttering is a form of disclosure and is described in more detail below.

Voluntary Stuttering

'Voluntary stuttering' is a treatment technique that has been a central feature of stuttering management for many decades. This procedure originated from the

Negative Practice techniques introduced in the 1930s and was written about extensively in the 1970s (Bloodstein, 1975; Dunlap, 1932; Van Riper, 1973).

Voluntary stuttering, also known as pseudo-stuttering, involves the speaker stuttering on purpose. The voluntary stutter should be produced slowly and deliberately for it not to turn into an uncontrolled stutter. Generally, only relaxed repeated movements should be used in voluntary stuttering. Fixed posture type stuttering may increase muscular tension and promote more stuttering, therefore should be avoided. Voluntary stuttering has two key benefits: (1) it serves as an obvious way to advertise stuttering early in a conversation and (2) voluntary stuttering is a primary technique in desensitisation of stuttering. The concept is that what a person can do deliberately should not be feared. For instance, a 30-year old client at the University of Utah Intensive Stuttering Clinic used voluntary stuttering during a job interview and reported it decreased his anxiety significantly.

Eye Contact

Within many cultures, maintaining appropriate eye contact during a conversation is important. In North America and most of Europe, making eye contact is interpreted as showing interest in your conversational partner and is a sign of self-confidence. People who stutter often communicate their embarrassment and negative reactions to their stuttering through poor eye contact. This, in turn, can make a listener feel uncomfortable, potentially increasing discomfort for both conversational partners. For the stuttering person, maintaining eye contact – especially during a moment of stuttering – lets a conversational partner know that they are in control of their conversation turn, are not embarrassed by the stuttering moment, and value the communication that is taking place (Breitenfeldt & Lorenz, 1999; Webster & Poulos, 1989). However, it is essential to consider that eye contact norms vary significantly around the world. In many parts of Asia, Africa and Latin American, only very brief eye contact is deemed acceptable.

A first step in improving eye contact is maintaining eye contact with oneself while talking in front of a mirror. After the client feels comfortable maintaining eye contact with themselves, treatment transitions to increasing eye contact with different conversational partners. When speaking to a group, it may be helpful for some speakers to direct the conversation to two or three people and maintain eye contact with those individuals. Other techniques include deliberately noting everyone's eye colour and consciously observing the reactions of listeners.

Cognitive Behaviour Therapy

Many adults and adolescents who stutter develop a set of adverse reactions to their stuttering. Stuttering management therapy may also involve elements of cognitive behaviour therapy (CBT) to address this problem (see also Chapter 6). The goal of CBT is to reduce social avoidance and fear (Craig & Tran, 2006; Menzies et al., 2009). The basic premise of CBT is that cognitions influence emotional reactions and behaviour. A process of cognitive restructuring can promote improved self-control and improved self-concept. Improved control can likewise lead to decreased feelings of self-doubt, shame and fear related to stuttering.

The core component of CBT for people who stutter is challenging unhelpful beliefs about possible negative evaluations by others (Rowley, 2012). CBT therapy comprises sessions where negative thoughts related to stuttering and social interaction are systematically modified. The first step is for the client and therapist to identify patterns of unhelpful thoughts. In the context of stuttering, evaluating negative thoughts may be accomplished through multiple means: (1) Individual counseling involving 'reframing' negative thoughts and emotions, (2) group problem-solving discussions related to anxiety management, (3) systematic desensitisation of stuttering fears by using disclosure and voluntary stuttering.

Modifying Moments of Stuttering

Stuttering modification approaches have the goal of lessening the severity of stuttering moments when they occur. In this respect, stuttering modification techniques are more reactive compared to the proactive management strategies listed above (Blomgren, 2009). Purposefully terminating a stuttering moment and canceling a stuttered word are reactive because the speaker uses the techniques to react to a moment of stuttering after it has already begun. Modifying a moment of stuttering can help a stuttering speaker regain control over a stuttering moment and recalibrate their speech system before moving forward. Stuttering modification techniques include (1) purposefully terminating a stuttering moment and (2) cancellation.

Terminating a stuttering moment is often referred to as a 'pull out.' It is used when the speaker becomes significantly 'stuck' on a particular sound and pulls out of the stuttering moment. It is most commonly used for fixed posture type stuttering moments rather than repeated movements. The speaker purposefully modifies the stuttering moment by relaxing the stuck speech articulators – the lips, tongue, or vocal folds. For example, a 20-year-old client, Daniel, was taught to identify moments where his articulators became fixed (stuck) during a stuttering moment. We had Daniel speak in front of a mirror to aid in determining the site of tension. After accurately identifying the area of muscular tension associated with stuttering moments, he practised gaining control over the stuttering by purposefully relaxing his tense articulators. Initial practice involved having him stutter on purpose (pseudo stuttering) and then consciously pulling out of the moment of stuttering.

Cancellation refers to saying a stuttered word again, ideally with decreased muscular tension. The stuttered word is repeated slowly and gently. The client 'cancels' the stuttered word with a fluent word. When a stuttered word is cancelled, the client is restabilising, or resetting, their speech system. Ideally, this would occur with the client simultaneously using a fluency facilitating technique like prolongation, gentle vocal onset, or starting the word with reduced articulatory pressure (see below).

The steps to a cancellation involve completing the stuttered word and stopping immediately. The client should not backtrack or repeat any other words than the one in which the stuttering occurred. The client should pause for 1 second, then begin the stuttered word again with a prolonged initial sound or reduced articulatory pressure. If stuttering occurs again during the cancellation attempt, the client should move on. Not all cancellation attempts will be successful, and the client should never feel that an unsuccessful cancellation is a failure of any kind.

Speech Restructuring Approaches

Speech restructuring refers to speech therapy where a client is taught to use a new speech pattern in all speaking instances. This approach contrasts with stuttering modification, where the focus is on addressing the stuttering moment. Slowed or prolonged speech is typically the primary component of any new speech pattern. The person who stutters may also be taught to produce their speech with less articulatory pressure and initiate vocal fold vibration in a gradual and controlled manner. These techniques are based on findings that stuttering speakers often use speech production strategies outside their speech motor control abilities.

Some speech restructuring approaches focus exclusively on speech rate reduction, and the specific techniques are often referred to as 'stretched syllables,' 'controlled rate,' or 'smooth speech' techniques. Other speech restructuring approaches combine prolonged speech with additional fluency-enhancing techniques (Blomgren, 2009; Boberg & Kully, 1985; Kroll & Scott-Sulsky, 2010; Webster, 1982). Speech restructuring therapy is an evidence-based approach to helping people who stutter improve their control over their speaking mechanism.

A common complaint of some speech restructuring therapies is the resulting speech may sound unnatural or 'robotic.' This adverse outcome may indicate that the client didn't adequately learn the techniques or that speech naturalness wasn't a focus of the treatment. It is critical for the techniques to be practised and integrated into the client's natural sounding speech pattern. That said, by design, using speech restructuring skills will result in a slightly different speech pattern than the client used before. Many stuttering speakers embrace this speech change process, but it may be uncomfortable or unnecessary for others.

Prolonged Speech

Prolonged speech is the primary fluency facilitating technique in nearly all speech restructuring therapies (Andrews et al., 1980). The prolongation of speech sounds results in increased control over the movements of the speech articulators. There are many approaches to prolonging speech production, from relatively simple to complex. Decreasing speech rate is best achieved by stretching the duration of sounds and syllables.

The most straightforward technique is to prolong the initial speech sound of each utterance. This initial utterance prolongation acknowledges that most stuttering occurs at the beginning of words and utterances. Using this approach, only the initial speech sound is stretched, while the remaining sounds and words are produced at a normal speaking rate. The prolonged sound should be produced with a light contact – no excess tension in the lips, tongue and larynx. Initially, the length of the prolongations should be exaggerated so that the client feels in control over their production. With practice, the duration of the initial prolongation may be shortened, but only if the client retains the feeling of control over their speech.

Other prolongation strategies involve more extensive utilisation of a prolonged speech pattern. For instance, the prolonged speech techniques used in the Stuttering Treatment Center at the Hollins Communications Research Institute in Roanoke, Virginia (Webster, 1982; Webster, 1986) and the University of Utah Intensive Stuttering Clinic (UUISC) (Blomgren, 2009) involve stretching the duration of all syllables. This 'slow motion' speech allows individuals to notice and alter their speech sound production, resulting in reduced force and abruptness of articulatory movements.

In the more intensive prolongation approach, speech is initially produced at a very slow rate. For instance, in the UUISC, all syllables are initially produced at a rate of 2-seconds per syllable. Speech rate is monitored with an analog stopwatch and a computer system specially designed to provide speech rate biofeedback. After fluent speech has been established at 2 seconds per syllable, syllable durations are systematically shortened to 1 second per syllable, half-second and finally to a 'controlled normal rate.' The controlled normal rate is where a person who stutters can speak with little or no stuttering while sounding as natural as possible. The final rate varies for each client, depending on their level of control. At all times, however, the client should produce speech as close to their natural speaking pattern as possible. It is unlikely a client will habituate their new speaking pattern into everyday life if they don't feel it sounds natural.

Gentle Vocal Onset

Many people who stutter make some speech sounds with abrupt vocal onsets. That is, they initiate vocal fold vibration with too much force and muscular tension. This tension may lead to stuttering moments – particularly on words beginning with voiced sounds. The *gentle vocal onset technique* allows stuttering speakers to initiate vocal fold vibration in a controlled, precise and relaxed manner. The gentle onset technique is used on words that begin with vowels and voiced consonants.

The gentle voice onset technique is most beneficial when used at the beginning of utterance, and it is essentially a refined way of beginning a prolongation. The gentle onset technique should initially be practised in
combination with exaggerated sound prolongations. The steps to a gentle
onset are: (1) take a comfortable breath to ensure adequate air support, but not
so big as to increase muscular tension, (2) start exhaling and immediately feel
the vocal cords start vibrating very gently, (3) then gradually increase the
strength (loudness) of vocal cord vibration up to the level of normal speaking.

Reduced Articulatory Pressure

The reduced pressure technique refers to producing speech sounds – mostly
consonants – lightly and gently, with no muscular tension and no abnormal
build-up of breath pressure. The technique allows speakers to reduce articulatory pressure and smoothly transition from speech sound to the next in running
speech. The reduced pressure technique should initially be intopractised in
combination with exaggerated sound prolongations. The steps for the reduced
pressure target are to (1) take a comfortable breath and (2) immediately, upon
exhalation, begin producing the initial sound. There should be a light articulatory contact or reduced air pressure to begin the consonant.

Generalisation of Skills

It is crucial to remember that stuttering in adolescents and adults is a chronic
condition, and there is no 'cure' for stuttering. Therefore, all stuttering therapy
involves teaching compensatory strategies. This is true whether the methods
involve stuttering management or speech restructuring. That said, the methods
described above can significantly reduce the frequency or severity of stuttering
moments and improve the stuttering speaker's self-confidence and ability to
manage anxiety, embarrassment and shame related to stuttering.

Managing one's stuttering and producing speech with the fluency-enhancing
strategies outlined above can be very difficult. Therefore, the stuttering client
must practise all learned techniques in everyday speaking situations. Common
activities that promote generalisation of skills include giving speeches, talking on
a phone, introducing oneself and others, mock interviews and talking about
elements of effective conversation to improve confidence in speaking. Role
playing various speaking scenarios within the clinic setting may help transfer
learned skills to 'real-life' speaking situations. It is important to note a single
rehearsal is rarely enough to facilitate the successful transfer of skills to out-of-
clinic practice. Usually, many practise trials may be needed.

Summary

For adolescents and adults, stuttering therapy has conventionally focused on
either (1) teaching new ways to manage and deal with the stuttering or

(2) teaching new ways of speaking that facilitate fluent speech. It is now more common to combine these. Truly successful stuttering therapy will help people who stutter decrease the severity of their core stuttering behaviour and improve the emotional and cognitive challenges of the disorder.

References

Andrews, G., Guitar, B., & Howie, P. (1980). Meta-analysis of the effects of stuttering treatment. *Journal of Speech, and Hearing Disorders.* 45, 287–307. 10.1044/jshd. 4503.287

Bennett, E. M. (2006). *Working with People who Stutter: a lifespan approach*, Upper Saddle River, N.J.: Pearson Merrill/Prentice Hall.

Blomgren, M. (2007). Stuttering treatment outcomes measurement: Assessing above and below the surface. *Perspectives on Fluency and Fluency Disorders.* 17, 19–23. 10.1044/ ffd17.3.19

Blomgren, M. (2009). *University of Utah Intensive Stuttering Clinic Therapy Manual*, Acton, MA, Copley Custom Textbooks.

Blomgren, M. (2010). Stuttering treatment for adults: an update on contemporary approaches. *Seminars in Speech and Language.* 31, 272–282. 10.1055/s-0030-1265760

Blomgren, M. (2012). Review of the Successful Stuttering Management Program. In S. Jelcic Jaksic & M. Onslow (Eds.), The Science and Practice of Stuttering Treatment: A Symposium. Chichester, UK: John Wiley & Sons, Ltd.

Blomgren, M., Roy, N., Callister, T., & Merrill, R. (2006a). Assessing stuttering treatment without assessing stuttering? A response to Reitzes and Snyder. *Journal of Speech, Language, and Hearing Research*, 1423–1426. 10.1044/1092-4388(2006/104)

Blomgren, M., Roy, N., Callister, T., & Merrill, R. (2006b). Treatment outcomes research: A response to Ryan. *Journal of Speech, Language, and Hearing Research.* 49, 1415–1419. 10.1044/1092-4388(2006/102)

Blomgren, M., Roy, N., Callister, T., & Merrill, R. (2005). Intensive stuttering modification therapy: a multidimensional assessment of treatment outcomes. *Journal of Speech, Language, and Hearing Research.* 48, 509–523. 10.1044/1092-4388(2005/035)

Bloodstein, O. (1975). Stuttering as tension and fragmentation. In J. Eisenson, J. (Ed.), *Stuttering: A symposium.* New York: Harper.

Blumgart, E., Tran, Y., & Craig, A. (2010). Social anxiety disorder in adults who stutter. *Depression and Anxiety.* 27 (7), 687–692. 10.1002/da.20657

Boberg, E. & Kully, D. (1985). *Comprehensive Stuttering Program: client manual.* San Diego, Calif.: College-Hill Press.

Breitenfeldt, D. H. & Lorenz, D. R. (1999). *Successful Stuttering Management Program (SSMP): For adolescent and adult stutterers*, Cheney, WA: Eastern Washington University Press.

Craig, A. R. & Tran, Y. (2006). Fear of speaking: Chronic anxiety and stuttering. *Advances in Psychiatric Treatment.* 12, 6. 10.1192/apt.12.1.63

Dunlap, P. K. (1932). *Habits: Their making and unmaking.* New York: Liveright.

Gabel, R. M., Hughes, S., & Daniels, D. (2008). Effects of stuttering severity and therapy involvement on role entrapment of people who stutter. *Journal of Communication Disorders.* 41, 146–158. 10.1016/j.jcomdis.2007.08.001

Healey, E. C., Gabel, R. M., Daniels, D. E., & Kawai, N. (2007). The effects of self-disclosure and non self-disclosure of stuttering on listeners' perceptions of a person who stutters. *Journal of Fluency Disorders.* 32, 51–69. 10.1016/j.jfludis.2006.12.003

Kraaimaat, F. W., Vanryckeghem, M., & Van Dam-Baggen, R. (2002). Stuttering and social anxiety. *Journal of Fluency Disorders*. 27, 319–330. 10.1016/s0094-730x(02)00160-2

Kroll, R. & Scott-Sulsky, L. (2010). The Fluency Plus Program: An integration of fluency shaping and cognitive restructuring procedures for adolescents and adults who stutter. In B. Guitar & R. Mccauley (Eds.), *Treatment of Stuttering: Established and Emerging Interventions*. Philadelphia: Wolters Kluwer / Lippincott Williams & Wilkins.

Lee, K. & Manning, W. (2010). Listener responses according to stuttering self-acknowledgement and modification. *Journal of Fluency Disorders*. 35, 110–122. 10.1016/j.jfludis.2010.04.001

Menzies, R. G., O'Brian, S., Onslow, M., Packman, A., St. Clare, T. & Block, S. (2008). An experimental clinical trial of a cognitive-behavior therapy package for chronic stuttering. *Journal of Speech, Language, and Hearing Research*. 51, 1451–1464. 10.1044/1092-4388(2008/07-0070)

Menzies, R. G., Onslow, M., Packman, A., & O'Brian, S. (2009). Cognitive behavior therapy for adults who stutter: A tutorial for speech-language pathologists. *Journal of Fluency Disorders*. 34, 187–200. 10.1016/j.jfludis.2009.09.002

Reitzes, P. & Snyder, G. (2006). Response to "Intensive stuttering modification therapy: A multidimensional assessment of treatment outcomes," by Blomgren, Roy, Callister, and Merrill (2005). *Journal of Speech, Language, and Hearing Research*. 49, 1420–1422; author reply 1423-6. 10.1044/1092-4388(2006/103)

Rowley, D. (2012). Cognitive behaviour therapy. In S. Jelcic Jaksic & M. Onslow (Eds.), *The Science and Practice of Stuttering Treatment: A Symposium*. Chichester, England: John Wiley & Sons, Ltd.

Ryan, B. P. (2006). Response to Blomgren, Roy, Callister, and Merrill (2005). *Journal of Speech, Language, and Hearing Research*. 49, 1412–1414; author reply 1415-9. 10.1044/1092-4388(2006/101)

Smith, A. & Kelly, E. (1997). Stuttering: A dynamic, multifactorial model. In R. F. Curlee & G. M. Siegel (Eds.), *Nature and Treatment of Stuttering: New directions*. 2nd ed. Boston: Allyn and Bacon.

Teesson, K., Packman, A., & Onslow, M. (2003). The Lidcombe Behavioral Data Language of stuttering. *Journal of Speech, Language, and Hearing Research*. 46, 1009–1015. 10.1044/1092-4388(2003/078)

Van Riper, C. (1973). *The treatment of Stuttering*. Englewood Cliffs, N.J.: Prentice-Hall.

Webster, R. L. (1982). *Precision Fluency Shaping Program: Speech reconstruction for stutterers*, Roanoke, VA: Communications Development Corporation.

Webster, R. L. (1986). Evolution of a target-based behavioral therapy for stuttering. In G. H. Shames & H. Rubin (Eds.), *Stuttering Then and Now*. Columbus, OH: Merrill Publishing.

Webster, W. G. & Poulos, M. (1989). *Facilitating fluency: Transfer strategies for adult stuttering treatment programs*, Tucson, AZ: Communication Skill Builders.

8   Narrative Practice in Stuttering Therapy

Mary O'Dwyer and Fiona Ryan

When White and Epston published their book '*Narrative Means to Therapeutic Ends*' in 1990, they laid the foundation for developing Narrative Practice (NP) as an approach to problem solving within the context of family therapy. Their premise is that people possess the knowledge, skills and strengths to change their problem-based story to a preferred story that fits with a preferred identity, hopes and ambitions.

Applying aspects of NP (White & Epston, 1990; 1998; 2007) to working with people who stutter provides a way to explore how stuttering may become a problem-based story, and how it can be understood within the cultural knowledge and experiences of family stories. NP *disrupts* the problem-based story via the *externalisation conversation*[1], when the problem is objectified and separated from the person, creating an opportunity to recognise *alternative ways of being* and *of performing a preferred narrative*. At the core of this disruption is the process where clinician and client *excavate and elaborate* upon a clear understanding of the person's experience of the problem. Additionally, narrative conversations can be used to facilitate the *re-authoring* process, where the client is encouraged to develop stories about himself that are alternative or '*out of step*' with the problem-based story.

This case study of Adam (36 years) demonstrates how aspects of NP are used as part of a therapy programme for stuttering.

Clinicians' Story

Experience in working with people who stutter led the authors to reflect on how to influence change in cognitive and emotional aspects of stuttering when developing the Free To Stutter...Free To Speak (FTS...FTS) intensive therapy programme. The clients' freedom, choice and focus on their communicative competence are cornerstones of this 6-day programme. By incorporating NP in therapy, these concepts are linked to *meaning-making* in personal narratives, along with taking action in the direction of *preferred identity* (Ryan, O'Dwyer, & Leahy, 2015). In addition to NP, aspects of stuttering modification and mindfulness are the main therapeutic elements employed.

DOI: 10.4324/9781003179016-8

Concurrent with the development of this programme, the authors participated in the European Clinical Specialization in Fluency disorders programme – an experience that challenged, encouraged and validated our exploration of innovative approaches that focus on the social model of intervention.

We adopt Van Riper's definition of stuttering (1971; p. 2), elaborating upon it, proposing that a person's reactions may include a central role of narrative in stuttering, i.e., *that the speaker develops a sense of self-who-stutters resulting from attributing meaning to personal experiences through self-narrative* (O'Dwyer, Walsh, & Leahy, 2018). The construction of self-who-stutters is influenced by the speaker's relationships. The narratives of people who stutter are key environmental factors contributing to causative epigenetic processes. Therapy seeks to highlight how *meaning-making* around experiences plays its part in the onset and development of stuttering, including its variability. This process involves discourses and stories including self-narratives, some of which are presented here as part of Adam's case study.

Narrative Practice during the FTS...FTS programme

NP conversations are scheduled daily within a small group of 2–3 participants, a clinician and a student clinician. Additionally, NP is also embedded in group reflections and discussions occurring outside of group work e.g., during meals and breaks. One key aspect of NP on the programme is the therapeutic use of documents, when written documents such as letters, emails and narrative maps are used. These documents further develop the re-authoring process, therapeutically increasing its impact significantly (Epston, 1998; 1999). They are used to supplement the face-to-face sessions by providing a permanent record of key moments highlighting unexpected nuances that can subtly shift the conversation and extend the context for clients. As they are tangible and can be re-read, documents can remind people how their stories change over time, giving a sense of history and highlighting points for reflection and possible future lines of enquiry. They may raise further questions about the working of the problem to develop a rich description, or may recall something particular the client said that the clinician wishes to question further. The use of documents in this way encourages the process of reflection both on the session and the narrative itself, serving to thicken the new preferred story. At the end of the intensive residential week, each person on the course is given a photographed copy of all their narrative maps as part of their own records and remembrances. These maps are added to the folders of informational material, artwork and supporting documents collated by the people attending the programme.

Adam's Story

Adam has a family history of stuttering, has stuttered since childhood, and had attended therapy previously. Married with three children, he has a responsible and satisfying job and describes his life as not confined in any major restrictive sense. However, Adam reports that every so often when contributing to a discussion at work 'I would pull back and say nothing, for fear of stuttering'. His stuttering involves repeating syllables, blocking with obvious tension, eyes closed momentarily. Adam states that his main ambition in attending therapy is to achieve acceptance. He writes: 'I don't like the suppression I give myself when I have the urge to say/comment in a conversation and I stop myself from expressing myself for fear of stammering, blocking'.

During group discussions, clinicians focus on problem talk in the initial days, objectifying the problem by referring to it in the words of the person who stutters – e.g., as 'the fear', 'the blocking' – thereby separating the problem from the person. Adam identifies and names his problem 'Stutts'. He is facilitated (Table 8.1) in providing a rich description of the effects of 'the Stutts' in his life, across various domains including family and work as well as his own self-esteem. Then, Adam is asked to take a position in relation to 'the Stutts'. This is an important moment in any externalisation conservation as it is often a light-bulb moment when the client understands and becomes aware that they are not the problem and that they have agency over the problem. The language used in objectifying the problem creates a sense of distance between the person and problem. This separation of person and problem then allows for the person to have an opinion and to make a choice about how they want their problem to change.

Externalising Conversations with Adam

A summary of the more formal externalisation conversation within Adam's small group is presented in Table 8.1. Adam describes that while 'Stutts' is

Table 8.1 Adam's completed statement of position map 1 (read from bottom up)

Category of Enquiry	Adam's Response
Hopes/Values Why?	I would rather see myself as a stutterer and continue to change it, but I will still be the stutterer. It's not just me, it's part of who I am.
Position: where do you stand on this?	Not pleased (with 'Stutts'). I have to put the hard work in. To become comfortable sometimes being stressed
Effects across domains of living	Has made many appearances at important stages in life. I don't let ('Stutts') meet family or friends. Like making speeches at graduation, college presentations, interviews and all the big stuff. As an embarrassment, something to avoid. Shamed me. Would be some low self-esteem.
Characterisation of problem/naming	'Stutts'. Since about seven or eight (years of age) and we've been more or less hanging around since then: Most of the time, something to control, something not to be embraced.

almost ever-present, he tries to conceal it even from family and friends. This leads to avoidance and negative emotional reactions and thoughts as Adam tries to control the problem. Leaving his 'work speak for itself' was comfortable for Adam. He identifies that normally he would shrug his shoulders, and was not a person who would express his opinion.

As this externalising conversation was taking place, Adam was also processing watching Alan Rabinowitz on DVD describe his stuttering as a 'gift' (Rabinowitz, 2005) (see also Chapter 9). He became upset at hearing stuttering referred to as 'a gift' and rather than say nothing, he spoke out about his response the following morning in group, having reflected on it and written in his journal the night before. This 'speaking out' was a turning point for Adam and helped identify 'the absent but implicit' which White (2000) discusses as an entry point into an alternative story. While Adam is speaking out about his difficulty with viewing stuttering as a gift, he is accessing what was implicit in that for him: that he might have but did not want to reject 'self-who-stutters'. What was absent but implicit was how he valued 'self-who-stutters'. This step of talking about stuttering as a gift or otherwise was identified as a unique outcome and an exception and was named 'speaking out'.

Externalisation conversations are composed of two landscapes, one of action (the plot or material of the story) and one of identity (what we think, know or feel). Narrative questioning addresses both the events and the meaning ascribed to those events (O'Dwyer & Ryan, 2020). Using questioning which focuses on the links between identity and action, the clinician asks if speaking out was his normal way. In this way, this new story line is extended, embedding it in to past actions (distant past and near past) with a view to spreading it into the present and opening up the possibility of future actions.

Figure 8.1 below presents a summary of part of this conversation focusing on the present step and what it made possible for Adam in the future. In this type of conversation, the clinician first focuses on naming the step or action that the client has taken. When named, focus shifts on to questions such as 'What does this mean for you?'; 'What does taking this step say about you?'. Then in order to 'historicise' this step, questions such as 'Can you tell me about a similar step you have taken in the past?' are asked. This is to ensure that the client sees the core step as linked to who they are/want to be and not a once-off/fluke happening. The conversation then moves to what this step makes possible for the person in the future, again linking action with identity.

Re-authoring Conversations

The development of the new preferred story begins with this alternative story line that emerged from identification of the unique outcome. The clinician asks Adam for other examples of him speaking out and Adam talked about an interview:

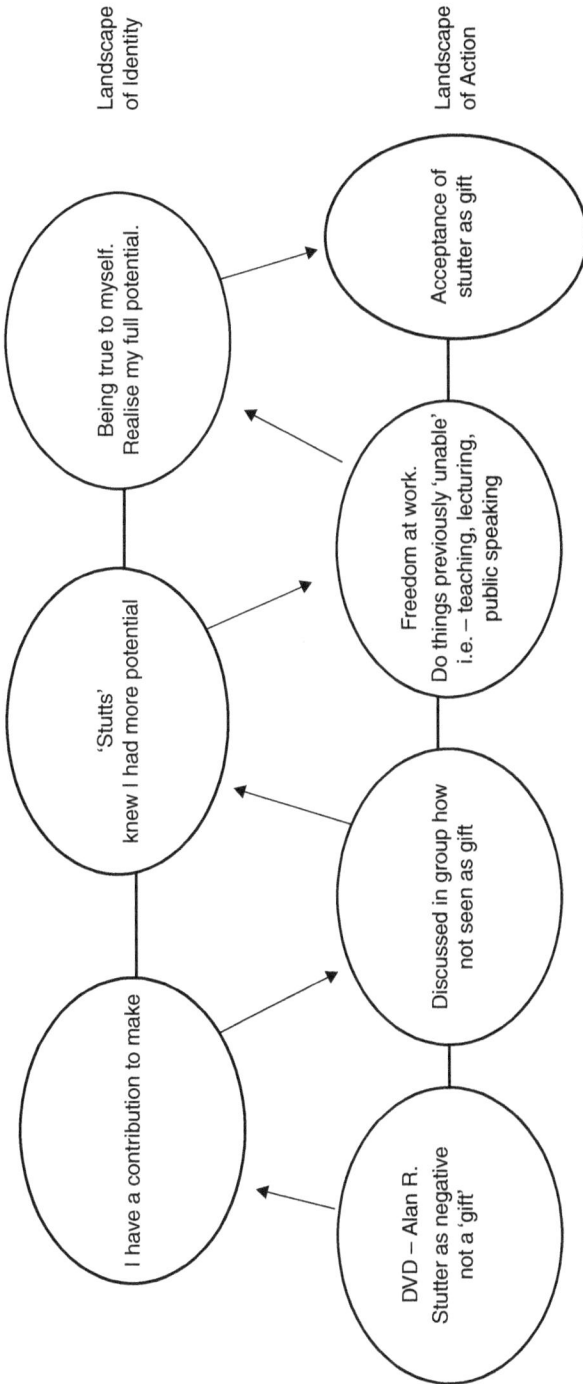

Landscape of Identity

Landscape of Action

Being true to myself. Realise my full potential.

Acceptance of stutter as gift

'Stutts' knew I had more potential

Freedom at work. Do things previously 'unable' i.e. – teaching, lecturing, public speaking

I have a contribution to make

Discussed in group how not seen as gift

DVD – Alan R. Stutter as negative not a 'gift'

Figure 8.1 Resisting the problem story – Adam.

> 'The interview went well. I received my results. I was pleased. It was one of the happiest days of my life. Through all of my books, drawings, I was able to convey all of my projects to someone I had not met. It was one of the most pleasant chats I've had. I was delighted to be able to communicate some of my ideas to a stranger.'

This further example linked (Adam identified the step as preparation) to the previous step of speaking out. The clinician then elicited the value Adam attributed to the step:

Clinician: 'and it was important to you to?'
Adam: 'to succeed.'
Clinician: 'so succeeding would be, in terms of identity, important?'
Adam: 'very important'

As the process continued Adam linked succeeding with overcoming hurdles including a change in roles wherein he became the house parent as his wife worked.

Adam: 'it is a balance in that, frustrated in being at home, frustrated that I spent so long in College that I chose this. It's a gift. Being able to spend so much time with the children'.

Adam reflected on the importance of 'giving back' because 'when you give something back you are rewarded'. Linking the steps taken together, the clinician asked:

Clinician: what are the steps taken? Right up to now, in the past, right up to now to the current steps.
Adam: I suppose I made a step Sunday night seeing opportunities. I am capable of more if I want to take that on.
Clinician: how would you name that step you took Sunday night?
Adam: mmm, is it too profound to call it an awakening?

Recognising the new story, Adam acknowledged difficulties he had with accepting himself as a person who stutters. He linked 'speaking out' with 'staying with it'. He needed 'to stick with it' to embrace his stuttering and himself as a person who stutters.

Table 8.2 summarises some of the key meanings that Adam linked to the step of 'speaking out'. It is important to stay with the language used by the client. For example the clinician suggested persistent as the key value taking her lead from Adam but he chose 'staying with it'. The conversation held was:

Adam: I do have that, persistant nature. I will stay with something,
Clinician: so persistent, is that the word?
Adam: well, persistent in a job that has to be done, if it takes two days or 2 years. I just stay at it.

Table 8.2 Adam's statement of position map 2 (read from bottom up)

Category of Enquiry	Adam's Response
Justifying the evaluation; Intentional understandings of this experience and understandings of what is accorded value (Why was this important for you, what does it tell me about what you value?)	I will **stay with** something, I just stay at it.
Evaluating effects of action/unique outcome **Experience of this development**	I was saying that in the journal, but then actually thinking about it. **I do it to something that has to be spoken about**, be it… Or whatever.
Effects of action/Unique outcome	That was a step. It brought out into the open, and the others said it could be this, could be that. They express their own opinions and I went away that evening, thought about it, **put my own twist on it** or whatever. The next day I talked about it, had a chat about it.
Characterisation of Initiative/ naming/describing the action/ unique outcome (What was the step you took that day?)	I just, **I spoke out.** I expressed an opinion.

Outcomes from Narrative Practice on the FTS…FTS programme

The relationship between unique outcomes (actions/times when the person's action contrasted with the problem story) and outcomes from narrative practice generally is documented by Matos et al. (2009). They identified two particular unique outcomes as important for therapeutic change: 1. Re-*conceptualisation:* where the client manifests thoughts and behaviours separate to the problem-dominated story, and understands the processes involved. 2. *New experiences:* described as new intentions, projects, activities or investments that are planned or in progress.

Evaluating outcomes of NP in the FTS…FTS programme involved 11 participants over a 3-year period. Ryan (2018) found that the impact of stuttering as measured by the Overall Assessment of the Speaker's Experience of Stuttering (OASES; Yaruss & Quesal, 2006) had decreased with statistical significance and this decrease was maintained over a 3-year period. Interpretative phenomenological analysis of the recorded sessions revealed rich themes linking narrative practice to reduction in the impact of stuttering and increased actions in everyday life, and a sense of enduring hope. As NP addresses the impact of stuttering, people take action, resulting in significant positive changes to quality of life, or indeed as the thoughts and feelings about stuttering undergo revision in NP, people are inspired to take action.

Pre-assessment OASES results were in the moderate range. Following the programme significant changes were noted across all subtests. Of note Adam's pre-programme OASES scores had been in the severe range for general information, 3 years following the programme, these scores remained in the mild range. Reactions to stuttering, quality of life and communications in daily situations also remained in the mild range 3 years after the programme.

However, it is of note that on one occasion Adam's OASES scores increased when his reactions to stuttering and communication in daily situations became mild–moderate before returning to the mild range. NP highlights that each story is subject to the development of rich subplots and developments. They are not linear, revision and reversals take place and the power of the original problem saturated narrative cannot be underestimated.

SSI-4 (Riley, 2009) results pre- and post-intervention are in the mild range with some slight decrease in score, highlighting that the observer's perceived severity or not, of stuttering behaviour is not always commensurate with the impact of stuttering on the person who stutters.

Outcome from Adam's Point of View

Participants were invited to respond to the results of the research described earlier. This is in keeping with the narrative process of documentation, inviting participants' response and engagement with the narrative process itself. Adam's response highlights the importance of the group in supporting the narrative process. He describes the busyness of his everyday life and the opportunity taken to tell his story after a lifetime of 'shutting myself up'.

> '*I was hopeful that something might happen. A Trigger, the magic Button!*
>
> *I don't know, it seemed like you looked like you could do it.*
>
> *There is energy to the group when the goal is one of positive action.*
>
> *I can't break it down better – but is must be that way – for within a short space of time, most, if not all the group, had opened themselves up. Definitely me anyway. I was, still am, keen to tell my story. Maybe that's because of an early life shutting myself up.*'

Adam's description of how narrative practice teases out the story highlights the impact of stuttering on his life and the importance of addressing impact within the therapeutic process.

> '*First session we open up. Egg cracking. The narrative therapy takes a hold. I began wondering, what's this, what's the magic, how's this work? You stop looking for answers and you hear the stories, you hear your story. It's teased out and brought along paths you may not have explored. But the crucial element is you*

participate in everyone's journey to here (FTS) and you see people's courage & look again at yourself & your journey & how your courage & your stutter has shaped you.'

NP highlights the importance of the stance taken by the clinician of curious partner unpicking the problem narrative rather than as an 'expert' professional passing judgement or making diagnoses.

Conclusion

NP has at its core an ethos of power sharing. Engagement with the narrative and the excavation of the problem is a joint endeavour between client and clinician. Adam's involvement in the narrative process results in awareness of the power of the stories we tell and hear about ourselves from early childhood on. For the clinicians, NP fits with the social model of intervention and within their own systems of practice. For Adam, NP resulted in a reduction of the impact of stuttering and increased participation in daily life.

Note

1 Italics used to denote terms specific to NP.

References

Epston, D. (1998). *Catching up with David Epston*. Adelaide: Dulwich Centre Publications.

Epston, D. (1999). Chapter 16: Co-Research: The making of an alternative knowledge (pp. 137–157). In *Narrative Therapy and Community Work: a conference collection*. Adelaide: Dulwich Centre Publications.

Leahy, M., O'Dwyer, M., & Ryan, F. (2012). Witnessing stories: Definitional Ceremonies in Narrative Therapy with adults who stutter. *Journal of Fluency Disorders*. 37 (0), 234–241. 10.1016/j.jfludis.2012.03.001

Leahy, M. & Warren, A. (2007). Making stuttering manageable: the use of narrative therapy. In: World congress on Fluency Disorders; Research, treatment and self-help in fluency disorders – new horizons; 320-324; 0955570018, 9780955570018

Matos, M., Santos, A., Goncalves, M., & Martins, C. (2009). Innovative moments and change in narrative therapy. *Psychotherapy Research*. 19 (1), 68–80. 10.1080/105033 00802430657

O'Dwyer, M., Walsh I. P., & Leahy, M. M. (2018). The role of narratives in the development of stuttering as a problem. *American Journal of Speech and Language Pathology*, 27 (3S), 1164–1179. 10.1044/2018_AJSLP-ODC11-17-0207

O'Dwyer, M. & Ryan, F. (2020). Narrative practice: Identifying and changing problem stories about stammering. In Stewart, T. (Ed.), *Stammering Resources for Adults and Teenagers*. London: Speechmark.

Rabinowitz, A. (2005). Keynote address at the Stuttering Foundation Annual Conference. Available to download @ The Stuttering Foundation (vhx.tv)

Riley, G. D. (2009). *SSI4 Stuttering Severity Instrument* (4th Edition). Austin Tx: ProEd.

Ryan, F. (2018). Stories from the other side: outcomes from Narrative therapy for people who stutter. Unpublished thesis.

Ryan, F., O'Dwyer, M., & Leahy, M. M. (2015). Separating the Problem and the Person. *Topics in Language Disorders*. 35 (3), 267. 10.1097/TLD.0000000000000062

Van Riper, C. (1971). *The nature of stuttering*. New Jersey: Prentice Hall.

White, M. (2007). *Maps of narrative practice*. New York: W.W. Norton.

White, M. (2000). *Reflections on narrative practice*. Adelaide: Dulwich Centre Publications.

White, M. & Epston, D. (1990). *Narrative means to therapeutic ends*. New York: Norton.

Yaruss, J. S. & Quesal, R. W. (2006). Overall Assessment of the Speaker's Experience of Stuttering (OASES): Documenting multiple outcomes in stuttering treatment. *Journal of Fluency Disorders*. 31 (2), 90–115. 10.1016/j.jfludis.2006.02.002

9 Dysfluency Studies: Rewriting Cultural Narratives of Stammering

Maria Stuart

The sstuttering is the most honest part of me

It is the only thing that never lies

It is how I know I still have a voice

I am still being heard

I am still here

When I stutter I am speaking my own language fluently

When I sound like this, I know my loved ones can find me

This is what I sssound like when I speak for myself

This is what I sound like

This is what I sound like.

(from 'Honest Speech', Erin Schick)[1]

This chapter explores the emerging field of Dysfluency Studies, an inter-disciplinary approach to stammering that is rooted in the humanities but in dynamic conversation with clinical practice. With its origins in work by cultural and literary scholars (Shell, 2005; Eagle, 2013; 2014), this inter-disciplinary perspective has developed through the Wellcome-funded re-search network 'Metaphoric Stammers and Embodied Speakers (MSES): connecting clinical, cultural and creative practice in the area of dysfluent speech' (2019). Encompassing researchers in the humanities, clinicians and creative artists, the network expands a clinical understanding of 'dysfluency' to incorporate its use and resonance across literary texts, cultural studies, film, music and visual arts. This chapter will use the ongoing work of the MSES network to illustrate the main features and core values underlying Dysfluency Studies and to explore how these could be harnessed to inform and support ongoing innovations in clinical practice.

Many of us in the MSES network have a personal experience of stammering which informs our research and our practice, and those involved approach

DOI: 10.4324/9781003179016-9

stammering not as a 'disorder' to be 'fixed' but as a form of communication that offers unique insight into the relationship between vocal agency and cultural reception – that intricate dynamic between what we say and how it is received. In the words of a recent publication in the field, *Stammering Pride and Prejudice* (2019) 'difference' is not 'defect' and our approach challenges a medically inflected model of 'recovery' premised on concepts of 'normal' speech and the pathologising of vocal difference. Instead, we explore the spaces opened up by dysfluency in terms of the richness, diversity and complexity of communication – the expressive resources, critical insights and communicative skills that come directly from the embodied experience of stammering. Drawing on the insights of Disability Studies (St Pierre, 2013), Dysfluency Studies foregrounds the role of the humanities in identifying and challenging the complex, often disabling cultural narratives around stammering. Crucially, it also foregrounds the power of creative writers, artists and musicians to subvert concepts of 'normative' speech through the power and potential of an expressive, generative dysfluency.

Drawing on a range of voices in the field, the chapter will explore the following questions:

- What is a speech 'disorder'? Is this an appropriate term for dysfluent speech? How might clinical practice resist and challenge a social regime of fluency?
- How do cultural representations of stammering both reflect *and* shape societal responses to dysfluency? How do these narratives impact on the lived experience of the person who stammers? How do they converge on the clinical encounter?
- In what ways can dysfluency be re-imagined in terms of vocal difference and diversity, as an experience that generates new understandings of the power relations, complexity and vitality of communication?

Beginnings

In 2005 Marc Shell published *Stutter* a landmark text that showed the possibilities for an interdisciplinary approach to dysfluency. As a scholar of comparative literature and one with a personal experience of stammering, Shell blended memoir with literary and cultural studies to explore and challenge the assumptions that have coalesced around stuttering speech over time and across borders, tracing the shifting meanings of dysfluency within both cultural and medical practice. Although Shell's book remains a key intervention in the area, 2013-14 saw the publication of several books that marked the emergence of Dysfluency Studies as an identifiable field of research. In 2014 Chris Eagle published *Dysfluencies: On Speech Disorders in Modern Literature*, exploring the history of speech pathology as it is reflected in the work of several writers including Wilfred Owen, Virginia Woolf and Philip Roth. Eagle focuses on 'works of literature written after 1861 (or post-Broca), that is after the neurological view of both language and language loss begins to permeate the literary imagination' (p.11), exploring how this 'neurological turn' is both represented and contested in literary practice. Eagle also edited the collection *Literature, Speech Disorders and Disability: Talking Normal* (2013) which includes contributions on representations of stammering, aphasia, mutism and Tourette's Syndrome across a range of cultural forms from biblical sources to literature, film, television and comic books[2].

Included in the collection (Eagle, 2013) is an influential contribution by Joshua St. Pierre: 'The Construction of the Disabled Speaker: Locating Stuttering in Disability Studies', a piece that addresses the complex position of stammering within Disability Studies, the cultural forces that combine to construct and debilitate 'the disabled speaker' and, crucially, the significance of the economic systems within which we live, work and speak, to the 'devaluing' of dysfluency. For St. Pierre (2013), capitalist economies generate a commodification of speech in their demands for forms of smooth and speedy communication, a set of communicative 'norms' that service a particular economic model of time-efficient productivity. Under such systems, stammering speech 'wastes' time, a 'valuation' that shapes and underscores broader societal responses:

> *Bodies not capable of meeting expectations of pace and productivity are therefore disqualified from full participation not only in the economic sector but also in social situations [...] [P]articularly fitting is the instance of stuttering because stutterers lack not the ability to communicate, but the ability to communicate in the 'right' way and within the 'appropriate' amount of time. (p. 15–16)*

St. Pierre highlights the economic narratives that can impact so significantly on the lived experience of those who stammer – our sense of restricted career paths, of professional structures and expectations premised on fluency, and the material and psychological consequences of an alignment of fluent speech with social authority. While drawing on the social model of disability (which defines 'disability' not as inherent in physical or neurological difference, but in the social structures that fail to accommodate and support that difference), St. Pierre also addresses the complexity of this identification for many within the stammering community:

> *Many stutterers resist the term 'disabled' because of the associated stigma and the desire to be sensitive to those with 'real' disabilities, and the lack of literature in disability studies is surely an indication that stuttering is not prominently identified as a disability. Conversely, it has been demonstrated here that stutterers are disabled insofar as they suffer from marginalization within society. Being caught in that indefinite territory between disability and ability, the conception and treatment of stuttering is thus uniquely framed. (p.17–18)*

St. Pierre revisits the social model in a later essay (St. Pierre, 2019), harnessing Alison Kafer's political/relational model of disability' (Kafer, 2013) to develop a more nuanced framework within which to situate stammering speech:

> *To put the two pieces of the political/relational model together, stuttering can therefore be understood as a political category applied to certain neurodiverse and dysfluent bodies that describes not a biological truth of the body but a relationship between people and their social and communicative environments. To speak dysfluently is to speak more slowly than our society allows. It is to stretch, repeat and block on words. But this, in itself, is no pathology. When dysfluency is transformed into a pathology called 'stuttering', this tells us less about our bodies in themselves than it does about the relation between the social world and our bodies – what speech patterns our society finds acceptable and useful. (p. 14)*

Metaphoric Stammers and Embodied Speakers

Building on the momentum around interdisciplinary approaches to stammering, in October 2018 the first conference dedicated to Dysfluency Studies took place in University College Dublin. Entitled 'Metaphoric Stammers and Embodied Speakers' (metaphoricstammers.wordpress.com), the event brought together clinicians working with children, adolescents and adults who stammer, those in the humanities engaged with cultural representations of stammering, and artists using their creative work to explore and express their own experience of dysfluency. Although coming from a variety of perspectives, those attending shared a resistance to medical models of stammering as a 'disorder' to be fixed, seeking instead to challenge 'normalising' concepts of speech and the kinds of narratives that support those. The title 'Metaphoric Stammers and Embodied Speakers' also spoke to that difficult relationship between the embodied and the metaphoric stammer: how stammering is *experienced* by those who speak dysfluently and how the stammer is *used* metaphorically by a predominantly 'fluent' culture to talk about other things (usually forms of perceived blockage or breakdown, both personal and social). As Eagle (2014) writes:

> *[V]irtually without exception in modern literature, speech pathologies are 'diagnosed' metaphorically as the symptom of some character flaw such as excessive nervousness or weakness, or treated as a symbol for the general tendency of language toward communicative breakdown, ambiguity, [...] misunderstanding. (p. 11–12; see also Martin, 2015)*

This tension between embodied experience and cultural representation was explored across several conference panels on literary, dramatic and cinematic 'stammers', as was the potential to generate new narratives carving a space for vocal difference and diversity[3].

A key finding from the conference was the permeability of our disciplinary 'borders' (e.g., the way in which broader cultural narratives necessarily converge on the clinical encounter) and the potential for further strengthening of interdisciplinary connections. This development from *exploring* links to *connecting* practice fed into the Wellcome-funded MSES project (2019). Central to the project is a willingness to recognise the necessarily entangled nature of any interdisciplinary practice, especially one moving between the humanities and medical/clinical practice. In the words of two scholars in the medical humanities, Fitzgerald and Callard (2016):

> *We do not, as scholars from different disciplines, bring together our objects and practices to one another through a kind of free-trade agreement; rather we re-enter a long history of binding, tangling and cutting [across subject areas] within which the current moves towards integration are much more weighted than they might first seen. (p. 5)*

Strikingly Fitzgerald and Callard advocate a 'dynamic of entanglement' (p. 5) rather than the push towards integration so beloved of much interdisciplinary research. For those of us in the MSES project, this speaks to our recognition of the necessarily messy, overlapping nature of our field – the capacity of voice and speech to reverberate across so many disciplines, spilling over academic and creative borders in challenging but generative ways.

Recent Voices in Dysfluency Studies

While the work of the Wellcome network is ongoing, two recent publications have further expanded the reach of Dysfluency Studies. *Stammering Pride and Prejudice: Difference not Defect* (2019) is the collaborative work of two clinicians, Chris Constantino and Sam Simpson, and a doctor and activist within the stammering community, Patrick Campbell. In their introduction to the book (with contributors from a wide range of views and backgrounds), the editors highlight the importance of the social model of disability in challenging both the prejudice around stammering speech and in laying the foundations of stammering pride:

> *The nature of stammering, its variability and hideability, can make it more challenging to understand as disabling [...] Fluctuations in frequency of stammering may alter how disabled we feel; this may also be altered by the perceived and actual hostility of the speaking environment. A person who chooses silence because of fear of stigma, one who is silenced by their effortful blocks, and one who speaks but is ignored through prejudice are all disabled, albeit in different ways. (p. xxiv)*

The editors balance an awareness of the deeply individual aspects of stammering with an advocacy for collective action and communal pride. Defining stammering pride as a 'counternarrative to the dominant societal narrative around fluency' (p. xxvi), they too draw on Schick's performance poem 'Honest Speech' cited at the beginning of this chapter: '[Schick's] open, direct resistance to social norms and reframing of stammering as her "voice's greatest symphony" and "the most honest part of me" encapsulates the growing movement of stammering pride' (xxvi). Schick is also (with St. Pierre) one of the founders of *DidIStutter*.org, another site for transformative approaches to dysfluency.

Of particular importance to a chapter that speaks to clinical practice, are the contributions of both Constantino and Simpson as they reflect on their own practice as clinicians. In 'Stutter Naked', Constantino (2019) recounts the changes in his own experience of stuttering and highlights how familiar narratives of 'overcoming' dysfluency are profoundly lacking in appreciation of the inherent value of stuttering in and of itself:

> *I am now more able to openly and comfortably stutter. I can delight in the surprise of an unexpected stutter or find humour in a particularly goofy manifestation of one. These experiences have led me to see my stutter as a valuable part of myself, something that adds to rather than detracts from my speech. I still have moments of struggle and avoidance; the difference is that now I also have moments of joy and delight. (p. 214)*

In 'Looking Back, Looking Forward', Simpson (who does not stammer) traces the impact of the social model of disability on her own development as a clinician, her growing concern that aspects of therapy might work towards strengthening norms around 'acceptable' speech and endorsing a societal regime of fluency. Citing an earlier piece (on *didistutter.org.*), Simpson (2019) revisits the early impact of disability studies on her own work:

> *Engaging clients in conversations about the contrasting ways difference is understood in society and the different ways stammering can therefore be defined is central to my approach to therapy. I frequently witness how liberating an understanding of the social model can be as it shifts the focus away from 'what is wrong with me' to critically examining 'what is wrong with the broader system in which I live'. Being explicit and transparent about my philosophy of therapy also enables clients to make informed decisions about what they feel might be helpful at a particular point of time. There is no 'one size fits all' in stammering therapy, so offering a range of approaches and recognising that preferences change over time affords greater client autonomy. (p. 149)*

Simpson charts the resistance she has encountered from some in the profession still heavily invested in the medical model, but, more recently, the emergence of a growing network of fellow clinicians and activists working to transform cultural responses to stammering. 'Looking Back, Looking Forward' ends with a radical proposition:

> *I can see a transitional role for speech and language therapists in terms of challenging social- and self-stigma to support people who stammer to fulfil their educational,*

professional and personal dreams and potential. However, in the way that
people with dialectical speech differences are no longer considered to have disordered
speech [...], I also hope for a future where stammering therapy will no longer be
needed. (p. 157)

Conversations around the future direction of speech and language therapy, including those questioning therapeutic intervention, have been an integral part of MSES network, generating differences of opinion that are recognised and respected. What has emerged from the work of clinicians in the network is a sense of the clinical encounter as a profoundly collaborative space, one relinquishing traditional ideas of the clinician as 'expert' in favour of a person-centred approach that recognises the experience, expertise and agency of the person who stammers. Consequently, the aim of therapy is not fluency, but a broader, more nuanced exploration of an individual's sense of their own stammer and how they wish to address it. Therapy may involve exploring ways of negotiating blocks or reducing avoidance and self-stigma, but these are seen as choices (not as clinical imperatives).

March 2021 saw the publication of a special issue of the *Journal of Interdisciplinary Voice Studies* (*JIVS*) dedicated to Dysfluency Studies. The introduction (Stuart & Martin, 2021) returns to Eagle's analysis of the tendency of cultural narratives of stammering to 'diagnose' dysfluent speech as a sign of individual weakness, failure and/or neurosis, and asks:

If this is true of literary and cultural expression, how are such associations
of dysfluency with personal or moral failure mobilized? How can scholars in
the humanities converse with clinical practitioners about cultural expectations
concerning fluency? (p. 124)

The articles in the special issue offer different responses to that question: a history of speech pathology across nineteenth-century Britain, France and Germany (Hoegaerts, 2021); the popularity of a stammering character from the nineteenth-century American stage (McGuire, 2021); an analysis of the dysfluent voices of the Victorian séance in the poetry of Robert Browning (Martin, 2021); the present crisis for dysfluent speakers within a neo-liberal economy the privileges fast, fluent and 'efficient' modes of speech (St. Pierre, 2021); and how 'hearing-oneself-speak' enables a re-thinking of the therapeutic claims of Delayed Auditory Feedback devices such as *The SpeechEasy* (Rodness, 2021).

Creative Voices

The *JIVS* includes a section for creative artists in which JJJJJerome Ellis and Conor Foran use music and graphic art respectively to 'put aesthetic practices [...] into creative and critical tension with medical and therapeutic values regarding fluent speech' (p. 126). Highlighting the lack of critical attention to the significance of race to the experience/expression of dysfluency, Ellis (2021) explores his stammer through musical time and in relation to the experiences of African Americans in historical time:

> [I]f the disabled speaker risks losing a publicly acknowledged subjecthood by virtue of his inability to adhere to normalized communicative choreographies, how is this risk compounded when the disabled speaker is, like me, black in North America? (p. 225).

At the heart of Ellis's interweaving of historical trauma and contemporary crisis is the concept of 'the clearing', a generative space (and time) opened to both the dysfluent *and* the fluent through the *shared* encounter with the stammer – a space powerfully evoked in a recent recording of Ellis for the podcast *This American Life* (2020). As a profoundly inclusive metaphor for the encounter between the stammering and the non-stammering voice, 'the clearing' offers a transformative way of rethinking the rich variety of communicative encounters that structure our lives – personal, professional, clinical – in a way that accentuates the deeply relational aspect of speaking and being heard.

In graphic artist Conor Foran's work (2020; Foran, Stuart & Martin, 2021), *visualising* dysfluency takes centre stage as he creates a special font (*Dysfluent Mono*) to embody his experience of stammering. Using elongated letters, repeated letters and blank spaces, he 'visualises' the different ways we can block on a word, alert to both the shared dimensions of stammering speech and its deeply individual shapes and sounds (the elements of his font can be mixed in form and frequency to represent individual voices).[4] Although this is a visual representation of stammering enabling those who stammer to 'see' their voice in terms of aesthetic beauty, it is also a new 'narrative' of stammering – each letter telling the story of how a word is spoken, the process and the effort of speaking dysfluently.

The power of creative art not only to challenge existing narratives of dysfluency but to generate new ones, is also evident in the writing of Jordan Scott. Scott's 2008 poetry collection *blert* explores the embodied experience of stuttering – how the stutter feels in the mouth, on the tongue, in the thorax – and how its unpredictability disrupts and enriches the rhythms of speech. As with Schick's performance of 'Honest Speech', a crucial part of the expressive force of Scott's poetry is in his reading of his work, his stammer underscoring and animating the poetic dimensions of dysfluency.[5] His recent children's book (with illustrator Sydney Smith), *I Talk Like a River* (2021), is based on his childhood and the importance of his father's description of his voice as 'like a river', negotiating the pebbles and rocks in its path. His father's simile for his speech was crucial to Scott's rethinking of his voice as a natural process, as a valued part of a reimagined landscape of speech.

There are many ways in which the different, intersecting strands of Dysfluency Studies speak directly to clinical practice, offering alternative narratives and voices to gather into the therapeutic space – and to push beyond its borders. Given my own work in literary studies (2014), I'm particularly drawn to recent clinical innovations in narrative practice (see chapter 8) and the possibilities for exchange between literary understandings of narrative and the role of narrative within a clinical setting. Entangling clinical and cultural 'narratives' works to move us beyond the dichotomy of disabling cultural narratives and their counterpoint in narratives of triumph and recovery, pointing instead towards narratives that are more nuanced, open-ended and ultimately generative, narratives offering their readers (dysfluent and fluent) new vocabularies for stammering, new metaphors for communication.

Notes

1 The extract from 'Honest Speech' is printed with the permission of the author, Erin Schick. The full text of the poem is available in Campbell, Constantino and Simpson (eds.), *Stammering Pride and Prejudice: Difference Not Defect* (2019, pp.1–2). Crucial to a full appreciation of Schick's poem is her performance at the National Poetry Slam (2014) https://www.youtube.com/watch?v=j8XOyY54-Ew.
2 See also Jay Dolmage's *Disability Rhetoric* (2014) and Steven Connor's *Beyond Words: Sobs, Hums, Stutters and other Vocalisations* (2014).
3 See metaphoricstammers.com for conference programme.
4 See also *Dysfluent* magazine (Foran, 2020).
5 For a fuller discussion of the 'poetics of dysfluency' see Stuart (2014).

References

Campbell, P., Constantino C., & Simpson, S. (2019). Introduction. In Campbell, P., Constantino C., & Simpson, S. (eds.), *Stammering pride and prejudice: Difference not defect.* Guilford: J&R Press, pp. xxi–xxix.

Constantino, C. (2019). Stutter naked. In Campbell, P., Constantino, C., & Simpson, S. (eds.), *Stammering pride and prejudice: Difference not defect.* Guilford: J&R Press, pp. 213–223.

Dolmage, J. (2014). *Disability rhetoric.* New York: Syracuse UP.

Eagle, C. (ed.) (2013). *Literature, speech disorders and disability: Talking normal.* New York & London: Routledge.

Eagle, C. (2014). *Dysfluencies: On speech disorders in modern literature.* New York & London: Bloomsbury.

Ellis, J. (2021). The clearing: Music, dysfluency, blackness and time. *Journal of Interdisciplinary Voice Studies.* 5 (2), 215–233. 10.1386/jivs_00026_1

Ellis, J. & Cole, S. (2020). Time bandit. *This American Life.* 713, August 7. https://www. thisamericanlife.org/713/made-to-be-broken

Fitzgerald D. & Callard, F. (2016). Entangling the medical humanities. In *Edinburgh Companion to the Medical Humanities,* Edinburgh: Edinburgh UP, pp. 35–49. 10.26530/ oapen_613682

Foran, C (ed.) (2020). *Dysfluent.* 60 pp., https://www.dysfluentmagazine.com

Foran, C., Stuart, M., & Martin, D. (2021). 'Visualizing dysfluency': Interview with Conor Foran. *Journal of Interdisciplinary Voice Studies.* 5 (2), 235–251. 10.1386/jivs_00027_7

Hoegaerts, J. (2021). Stammering, stuttering and stumbling: A transnational history of the pathologization of dysfluency in nineteenth-century Europe. *Journal of Interdisciplinary Voice Studies.* 5 (2), 129–146. 10.1386/jivs_00021_1

Hooper, T. (2010). *The King's Speech* (DVD), UK: UK Film Council, See-Saw Films and Bedlam Productions.

Kafer, A. (2013). *Feminist, Queer, Crip*. Bloomington, IA: Indiana UP.

McGuire, R. (2021). *Our American Cousin*, our dysfluent nation: Transatlantic stammering on the nineteenth-century stage. *Journal of Interdisciplinary Voice Studies*. 5 (2), 147–162. 10.1386/jivs_00022_1

Martin, D. (2021). A warm and sympathetic thing: Voice and dysfluency in Robert Browning's 'Mr Sludge, "The Medium". *Journal of Interdisciplinary Voice Studies*. 5 (2), 163–178. 10.1386/jivs_00023_1

Martin, D. (2015). Stuttering in Victorian studies. *The Floating Academy*, https:// floatingacademy.wordpress.com/2015/05/05/stuttering-invictorian-studies/more-2776. Accessed 25 November 2016.

Martin, D. & Stuart, M. (eds.) (2021). Introduction, *Metaphoric Stammers and Embodied Speakers* (special issue on dysfluency). *Journal of Interdisciplinary Voice Studies*. 5 (2), 123–128. 10.1386/jivs_00020_2

Rodness, R. (2021). Stutter and phenomena: The phenomenology and deconstruction of delayed auditory feedback. *Journal of Interdisciplinary Voice Studies*. 5 (2), 197–213. 10.1386/jivs_00025_1

Schick, E. (2014). Honest speech. *Button Poetry*, National Poetry Slam https://www.youtube.com/watch?v=j8XOyY54-Ew

Schick, E. & St Pierre, J. (2014–21). *Did I Stutter*, www.didistutter.org/about.html. Accessed 13 May 2021.

Scott, J. & Smith, S. (2020). *I Talk Like a River*. New York: Neal Porter Books.

Scott, J. (2008). *blert*. Toronto: Coach House Books.

Simpson, S. (2019). Looking back, looking forward. In Campbell, Constantino & Simpson, (eds.), *Stammering pride and prejudice: Difference not defect*. Guilford: J&R Press, pp. 145–158.

St. Pierre, J. (2013). The construction of the disabled speaker: Locating stuttering in Disability Studies'. In Eagle, C. (ed.), *Literature, speech disorders and disability: Talking normal*. London: Routledge, pp. 9–23.

St. Pierre, J. (2019). An introduction to stuttering and disability theory: Misfits in Meaning'. In Campbell, Constantino, & Simpson (eds.), *Stammering pride and prejudice: Difference not defect*. J&R Press, pp. 3–18.

St. Pierre, J. (2021). Talking heads and shitting in the street: Stuttering *Parrhesia* in three modes. *Journal of Interdisciplinary Voice Studies*. 5 (2), 179–195. 10.1386/jivs_00024_1

Stuart, M. (2014). The poetics of dysfluency: Emerson and Dickinson. In Dillane, F., Stuart, M., & Sweeney, F. (eds.), *Maintaining a Place: Conditions of metaphor in modern American literature*. Dublin: UCD Press, pp. 29–46.

Stuart, M. (2019). Easy listening': Altered auditory feedback and dysfluent speech. *Journal of Interdisciplinary Voice Studies*. 4 (1), 7–19. 10.1386/jivs.4.1.7_1

Shell, M. (2005). *Stutter*. Cambridge, Mass.: Harvard UP.

10 An Adolescent with Cluttering

Susanne Cook and Charley Adams

Historical Background of Cluttering

The term 'cluttering' was likely coined in English by the British James Hunt in 1861 (Van Zaalen & Reichel, 2015). Weiss (1964) believed that cluttering was the 'verbal manifestation' of a Central Language Imbalance, the linguistic component of cluttering which clearly differentiates cluttering from stuttering. Bazin (1717) focused on the neurology of cluttering, noting that "this disturbance depends more upon the mind than upon the tongue" (in Weiss, 1964 p. 2), Colombat (1830) described a rapid speech rate and difficulties with word finding (in Weiss, 1964 p. 3), and Kussmaul (1877) observed that cluttering "improves when the patient pays attention to what he is saying" (in Weiss, 1964 p. 3). The success of Weiss' landmark text on cluttering would go on to ignite interest and research in cluttering in the United States (van Zaalen & Reichel, 2015), and culminated in the publication of "Cluttering: A Clinical Perspective" (Myers & St. Louis, 1996).

Definitions of Cluttering

Weiss (1964) defined cluttering as a disorder of speech "characterized by the clutterer's unawareness of his disorder, by a short attention span, by disturbances in perception, articulation and formulation of speech and often by excessive speed of delivery" (p.1). This lack of awareness and/or concern for their difficulties with speech was a common component of popularised definitions, however this component would begin to fade before the end of the twentieth century.

St. Louis and Schulte (2011) developed their 'lowest common denominator' definition:

> "Cluttering is a fluency disorder wherein segments of conversation in the speaker's native language typically are perceived as too fast, too irregular, or both. The segments of rapid and/or irregular speech rate must further be accompanied by one or more of the following: (a) excessive 'normal' dysfluencies; (b) excessive collapsing or deletion

DOI: 10.4324/9781003179016-10

of syllables; and/or abnormal pauses, syllable stress, or speech rhythm." (pp. 241–242).

In 2016, the International Cluttering Association formed an ad-hoc committee to develop an updated definition of cluttering that would be clear, concise, functional and consensus driven.

This committee stated that at the current point in time they were "in the formative – rather than conclusive – stage of establishing a definitive scientifically-based definition" (p. 1) and therefore developed the Three-Pronged Approach to the Conceptualization of Cluttering (TPA-CC, Myers, et al., 2018). The goal of the TPA-CC is not only to list observable symptoms, but also to hear and see the cluttering, and to provide experiential testimony from people who clutter and their loved ones. The International Cluttering Association (www.icacluttering.com) is in the process of gathering audio and video clips of cluttering, as well as testimony as described earlier, in order to provide a better understanding of cluttering. The three prongs to establish if someone presents with cluttering are (1) description of symptoms (see list below), (2) video and audio clips of cluttering and (3) testimony from people who clutter and their loved ones. The purpose of the testimony is to lend perspective to the outward behaviours of cluttering, including the potential psychosocial impact.

Symptoms and Subtypes of Cluttering

Symptoms of cluttering include the following: speech rate perceived to be too fast and/or irregular, speech dysfluencies which are not like typical stuttering dysfluencies, distortions and/or deletions of sounds and syllables, inappropriate prosody, poor topic maintenance, circumlocution and excessive revisions.

The effect of cluttered speech is that the listener must work harder to follow and understand. A more thorough description of cluttering symptoms, with examples (the complete TPA-CC), can be downloaded from the ICA website. People who clutter often report difficulty organising their thoughts cohesively, typically resulting in frustration on the part of the listener and the speaker.

Two distinct manifestations of cluttering have been identified: a) fast and unclear speech or b) difficulties with planning and formulating thoughts. Ward (2006) describes the first type as motoric cluttering, which Van Zaalen and Reichel (2015) label as phonological cluttering. The second type is described as linguistic cluttering (Ward, 2006) or syntactic cluttering (Van Zaalen & Reichel, 2015).

Case Study

This case study describes the case of 'Allen', a 16-year-old male diagnosed with cluttering. The assessment, diagnosis, therapy plan and treatment over 30 half-hour sessions is described in detail, including outcomes. Allen's parents reported concerns related to their son's speech fluency. During assessment, the therapist noted that Allen at times displayed a high rate of speech, including unintelligible segments, as well as unorganised responses with revisions. Additionally, Allen's handwriting was illegible, and he displayed some difficulties in social interactions, such as topic maintenance.

Cluttering Assessment

Predictive Cluttering Inventory (PCI)

The PCI (Daly, 2006) is a tool for assisting therapists in making differential diagnostic discriminations among (1) people who clutter, (2) people who both clutter and stutter and (3) those who do not have a fluency problem such as stuttering or cluttering. The instrument collects data in the areas of Pragmatics, Speech-Motor, Language-Cognition and Motor Coordination-Writing Problems. Under each category, descriptive statements are rated on a 7-point Likert scale ranging from "always" (6) to "never" (0).

Data from three adults familiar with Allen (one parent, two teachers) indicated a diagnosis of cluttering, and data from a fourth adult (teacher) indicated a diagnosis of both cluttering and stuttering. Poor motor control for writing, an irregular speech rate, confusing wording by rephrasing sentences and word-finding problems were significant. It was reported that Allen could get lost in details when retelling a story, and that he would rarely repair a communication breakdown. Allen's dysfluencies were mostly repetitions of words.

Speech Sample Analysis

A speech sample is used to examine language planning, and to calculate the mean articulatory rate (MAR). Following procedures outlined by Van Zaalen and Reichel (2015), the MAR is calculated using five fluent speech samples of between 10 and 20 syllables in length. During speech sampling, Allen was asked to talk about a topic of personal interest; he chose to talk about a video game. Allen's language planning seemed appropriate during this sample. His MAR of 6.7 syllables per second was significantly higher than the average rate for teenagers (5.5 syllables per second, see Van Zaalen & Reichel, 2015, p. 78).

Retelling a Memorised Story

During this task, the therapist reads a story to the client which contains main story elements and side issues. After listening, the client is instructed to retell the story as completely as possible to show the extent to which he or she is able to convey a message that someone else has already formulated. Allen was administered "The Wallet Story" (Van Zaalen & Reichel, 2015) which is a narrative with main story elements and side issues. Allen was able to recall 9 of the 13 main elements, and 4 of the 9 side issues. He added one detail that was not part of the original story. Allen was observed to rephrase mid-sentence five times, indicative of possible difficulties with language planning.

Screening Phonological Accuracy (SPA)

The Screening Phonological Accuracy (SPA) test (Van Zaalen et al., 2011) is designed to identify difficulties with phonological encoding. This assessment involves the repetition of several phrases containing multisyllabic words, and provides detailed information on accuracy, flow and syllable rate. Van Zaalen et al. (2011) defined accuracy as articulatory precision, and flow as the absence of pausing, telescoping and dysrhythmic speech. Allen displayed difficulties in the areas of pausing, sequencing of syllables and flow. His rate during this exercise was at 5.8 syllables per second, which shows that he was able to control his rate of speech during a structured situation. Allen's total score of 19.8 indicated a moderate disorder.

Psychosocial Impact of Cluttering

Even though Weiss (1964) described how people with cluttering show an indifference and lack of concern, the adverse emotional impact of cluttering has been widely documented (Bennett, 2006; Daly, 1986; Reichel, 2010), and affective responses can include anxiety, frustration, anger and sadness (Van Zaalen & Reichel, 2015). Van Zaalen and Reichel further mentioned the importance of addressing the cognitive and affective components of cluttering. Therefore, the psychosocial impact of Allen's fluency disorder was measured with the "Speech Questionnaire" (Cook, 2013). This paper-pencil questionnaire was designed to measure the health-related quality of life of children who stutter by asking 27 questions in the four categories of General knowledge, Feelings, Different speaking situations and Impact of stuttering". This valid and reliable questionnaire has been standardised for children and adolescents, aged 8;0 to 17;11 years. Allen's overall score of 64 indicated a mild to moderate impact of the fluency disorder on his life. Specific situations where Allen identified the greatest impact were speaking to adults, speaking on the telephone, making friends and doing the things he wants to do.

Results of the evaluation indicated that Allen presents with a cluttering disorder, characterised by a high rate of speech, as well as difficulties in overall speech accuracy, flow, pausing and telescoping. These difficulties impact his overall intelligibility in conversations with peers and adults. Allen also presented with some language planning difficulties, and a mild to moderate psychosocial impact of the fluency disorder on his life, specifically in the areas of speaking situations and making friends.

Therapy Plan

The complex symptomatology of cluttering requires a multi-dimensional therapy approach (Sick, 2014). Sick stated that the lack of evidenced-based studies does not mean that speech-language therapy is inefficient for cluttering (p. 124). Her suggestion was to develop a treatment plan which addresses those areas of concern that were identified during the evaluation process. For a multi-dimensional treatment approach, it is suggested to work on identifying cluttering symptoms, pausing, appropriate prosody, modification of speech and adapting to communicative demands, for example, focusing on the listener (see for example Sick, 2014, Van Zaalen & Reichel, 2015).

Allen's language planning was relatively cohesive, so the therapy plan targeted the phonological features of cluttering, with the following goals:

1   Identify and reduce the rate of speech during structured situations in phrases, sentences and structured conversation to a maximum of 5.8 syllables per second from the baseline of 6.7 syllables per second in at least 80% of opportunities.

   a   Identify the rate of speech in others and self with audio feedback and "live" in phrases, sentences and structured conversations.

   b   Achieve a MAR of a maximum of 5.8 syllables per second in phrases, sentences and in structured conversations.

2   Correctly produce 3–4 syllable words on word level, in phrases and in sentences with 80% accuracy:

   a   Correctly identify the number of syllables in multisyllabic words.

   b   Produce 3–4 syllable words with accurate sequencing of phonemes.

3   Recognise a communication breakdown by utilising learned strategies in at least 80% of opportunities.

   a   Allen will list indicators of misunderstanding by the listener (e.g., looks of confusion, response does not match the topic, no response from communication partner, etc.).

   b   With or without a checklist, Allen will recognise when he has been misunderstood (for example, confused look of the listener, answer does not match the topic, reaction of listener).

4   Clarify misunderstandings by utilising learned strategies (e.g., increase volume, slow down, speak clearly) in structured and unstructured situations with 80% accuracy.

   a   Allen will clarify misunderstandings during a structured conversation with the therapist.

   b   Allen will repair a communication breakdown during an unstructured speaking opportunity, such as in-vivo training.

Therapeutic Exercises

Allen was seen once per week for a total of 30 sessions in a one-on-one setting. Each session was 30 minutes long. The focus of the first 10 sessions was on awareness and identification. This included identifying the rate of speech in others and self, identifying place, manner and voicing of all phonemes; identifying the number of syllables in multisyllabic words; and listing the criteria for recognising a communication breakdown.

To simplify the identification of the rate of speech, the numbers 1 to 5, representing the range of speech rates, were introduced to Allen as follows:

1   Super slow-motion (comparable to a super slow-motion replay on TV during a sporting event)
2   Slow speech (comparable to speaking slower than normal)
3   Normal rate (the listener can understand everything easily)
4   Fast rate (the rate is fast, but still intelligible)
5   Super-fast rate (speech is unintelligible)

The clinician modelled the five different rates for Allen, and different speech samples were compared and rated accordingly. This rating method is both quick and accurate. Allen and the clinician decided that a rate between 3 and 4 is the goal, and a target rate of 5.8 syllables per second was agreed upon. After the introduction of the rating scale, the following hierarchy was used for the identification of speech rate:

1   Listen to audio/video samples of others and determine their rate of speech by rating it, and then calculating the MAR.
2   Listen to the clinician giving sentence examples and during a structured conversation and assigning a speed rating, and then calculating the MAR.
3   Listen to his own speech on a recording and rating it, and then calculating the MAR.
4   Identifying his rate of speech without having to listen to a recording.

Next, Allen and the clinician worked on identifying place, manner and voicing of all phonemes (see worksheet in online material). This is an important basis for increasing the kinesthetic awareness when producing speech. Following this, Allen worked on identifying the number of syllables in multisyllabic words. The clinician presented Allen with different words, 2 to 6 syllables in length, and asked him to identify the number of syllables in each word. One helpful strategy was clapping or tapping out the syllables, which is described in detail by Van Zaalen and Reichel (2015). The final task addressed during the identification phase was listing criteria for recognising a communication breakdown. If a listener does not understand a message, he or she might look confused, their answer might not match the topic, they might not answer at all or they might ask for a repetition. After listing these potential signs, identifying a communication breakdown was practiced with short, hypothetical scenarios.

The identification phase lays the foundation for the modification phase, and some of the identification exercises will carry forward into other exercises. Having spent the first sessions identifying cluttered features in others, the following ten sessions were focused on Allen identifying these features in his own speech. The first step was identifying his own rate in different situations. The goal was to have a rate of a maximum of 5.8 syllables per second. Initially, this was achieved by Allen rating on a scale how fast he thought he was speaking in recordings of short, structured conversations about a given topic. The clinician and Allen then calculated the rate of speech with PRAAT (Boersma & Weenink, n.d.), and compared it with his initial rating. This exercise helped Allen to learn to identify his own rate of speech with increasing accuracy.

To address self-identification with multisyllabic words, Allen was given word lists of 3- to 5-syllable words. First, slow motion speech was introduced as a method to help accurately sequence the phonemes in these words. Next, while being recorded, Allen was asked to generate a sentence with each of these words. As he listened to the playback, Allen had to determine if he articulated each syllable in the target words, without sequencing errors. When he had mastered that task, Allen was given reading material containing multisyllabic words. One focus was to achieve accurate articulation of the (initially highlighted) multisyllabic words, in addition to working on appropriate pausing and prosody. For this task, it was helpful for Allen to mark pauses and changes in prosody (e.g., raising the voice for a question, dropping the voice at the end of a sentence, etc.) in the text.

To further work on identifying a communication breakdown, Allen was asked to recognise signs of a communication breakdown (i.e., confused look of the clinician, answer did not match the topic, clinician asked for repetition, etc.) during speaking opportunities with increasing levels of linguistic complexity. Allen and the clinician then compiled a hierarchy of strategies on different ways to repair a communication breakdown: repeat the message, reword the message, slow down, speak clearly, say each syllable in the word. These repair strategies were practiced with the clinician and as homework with a parent.

The final ten sessions concentrated on focusing on the listener, and on generalisation of learned strategies in conversations with others. During this phase of therapy, Allen had to observe the listener to ensure that no communication breakdown occurred, and in instances where there were signs of a breakdown, he had to utilise a strategy to repair it. Again, exercises included situations with increasingly complex language, as well as increasingly difficult situations. This part of the therapy also included in-vivo training, and addressed Allen's identified impact of cluttering difficulties when speaking with others (such as speaking with adults, in front of a group of people and on the phone). The hierarchy of generalisation was: 1) role-play with the clinician;

2) in-vivo situation with support of the clinician; 3) generalisation with support from family; and 4) practice on his own and report back to the clinician.

Therapy Outcomes

After the 30 sessions, Allen could identify and reduce his rate of speech during structured speaking opportunities in 79% of measured situations. He further showed steady progress in articulating multisyllabic words with an average accuracy of 73% for identifying and monitoring the correct production of multisyllabic words. It was noted that he still required auditory feedback (recordings) in order to monitor his own correct production of these words in sentences or reading exercises. Allen could utilise different strategies to recognise and repair a communication breakdown when given one initial verbal prompt, or when using a visual with an average accuracy of 80%; during less structured situations his accuracy fell off slightly to around 71%.

Discussion and Conclusion

Although therapy had not yet addressed every aspect of Allen's cluttering identified during the evaluation, Allen and his parents chose to terminate therapy after 30 sessions because they were satisfied with his progress and ability to apply learned strategies across a variety of situations. Data showed positive trajectories for rate, self-awareness, clarity of speech for multisyllabic words, as well as for recognising and repairing communication breakdowns. This case study demonstrates how outcomes can be impacted by considering the perspective of the person who clutters, as well as that of the family (as stated in the TPA-CC, Myers et al., 2018). The affective component of Allen's cluttering was identified with the Speech Questionnaire and was addressed through the in-vivo-training. Allen reported after these in-vivo exercises that his nervousness dropped, and that he felt better about talking in these situations.

References

Bennett, E. M. (2006). *Working with people who stutter: A lifespan approach.* Upper Saddle River, N.J.: Pearson Merrill/Prentice Hall.

Boersma, P. & Weenink, D. (n.d.). *Praat: Doing phonetics by computer.* [online] Available at: https://www.fon.hum.uva.nl/praat/

Cook, S. (2013). Development of a questionnaire to determine psychosocial impact of stuttering for children and adolescents. *L.O.G.O.S. Interdiszplinär*, 21(2), 97–105. 10.7345/prolog-1302097

Daly, D. (1986). The clutterer. In K.O. St. Louis, (ed.), *The atypical stutterer: Principles and practice of rehabilitation.* New York: Academic Press, pp. 155–192.

Daly, D. A. (2006). *Predictive Cluttering Inventory (PCI).* [Online] Available at: https://drive.google.com/file/d/188NTu5Qz5iZ7wjgwxkR5g-y8s0MDxPfs/view [Accessed 11 05 2021].

Myers, F., Bakker, K., Cook, S., Reichel, I., St. Louis, K., & Van Zaalen, Y. (2018). *A Clinical Conceptualization of Cluttering*. [online] *icacluttering.com*. International Cluttering Association. Available at: https://sites.google.com/view/icacluttering/information/the-conceptualization-of-cluttering. [Accessed 11 05 2021].

Myers, F. L. & St. Louis, K. O. (1996). *Cluttering: A clinical perspective*. San Diego: Singular Pub. Group.

Reichel, I. K. (2010). Treating the person who clutters and stutters. In K. Bakker, L. J. Raphael & F. L. Myers (eds.), *Proceedings of the First World Conference on Cluttering*. Garden City NY: Adelphi University, pp.99–107. 10.13140/2.1.1588.7369

Sick, U. (2014). *Poltern. Theoretische Grundlagen, Diagnostik, Therapie*. Stuttgart: Thieme. Available at: 10.1055/b-0034-93463

St. Louis, K. O. & Schulte, K. (2011). Defining cluttering: The lowest common denominator. In D. Ward & K. Scaler Scott, (eds.) *Cluttering: A handbook of research, intervention and education*. East Sussex: Psychology Press, pp. 233–253.

Van Zaalen, Y., Cook, S., Elings, J., & Howell, P. (2011). *Screening phonological accuracy, effects of articulatory rate on phonological encoding*. Groningen, the Netherlands: Speech Motor Conference.

Van Zaalen, Y. and Reichel, I. (2015). *Cluttering: Current views on its nature, diagnosis, and treatment*. Bloomington, In: Iuniverse Inc.

Ward, D. (2006). *Stuttering and cluttering, Framework for understanding and treatment*. East Sussex: Psychology Press. 10.4324/9780203892800

Weiss, D. A. (1964). *Cluttering*. Englewood Cliffs, N.J.: Prentice-Hall.

11 Multicultural Commonalities in Stuttering and Intervention

Francesca Del Gado, R. Sertan Özdemir,
Selma Saad Merouwe, and Katarzyna Węsierska

Introduction

Cultural heritage has enormous influence on our lives. In fact, it shapes our beliefs, values and perspectives, as well as our way of thinking and our attitudes towards communication disorders (Shapiro, 2011). As clinicians, our duty is to listen to our clients and consider their cultural heritage through their eyes, including their ethnicity, religion and traditions (Turnbull et al., 2006). By listening to their personal histories, for example, we can learn to understand how the historical, geographical and social factors foster cultural attachment and identity, in addition to differentiating them from their ethnic group. By taking these considerations into account, we will communicate more meaningfully and enhance good therapeutic alliances with clients from different cultural backgrounds. Clinicians need to recognise both similarities among ethnic groups, and the individual differences within any group. Cultural values affect not only a community's assumptions about the aetiology of stuttering, the attitudes towards the phenomenon and towards individuals who stutter, but also how the community conceptualises therapy and its goals (Bloodstein et al., 2021). This chapter discusses multicultural considerations that usually influence the clinical process with clients and their families. It focuses on the commonalities and differences shared by four culturally diverse countries: Italy, Lebanon, Poland and Turkey. The Speech and Language Therapy (SLT) profession is established in all four countries, but levels of development and numbers of clinicians differ considerably between them.

Commonalities

The main commonalities among these four cultures are: certain misconstrued beliefs about the causes of stuttering; early responses to the beginning of stuttering; attitudes and social stigma; and a preference shown for fluency shaping approaches if seeking reduction or elimination of the disorder.

DOI: 10.4324/9781003179016-11

Knowledge about the Causes of Stuttering

Linking stuttering onset directly to a child's experience of trauma is a popular belief in all four societies, shared among parents and often by some professionals, including e.g., pediatricians, psychologists and teachers (Antoun & Saad Merouwe, 2018; Węsierska, et al., 2017). Such a traumatic event may be either physical (e.g., some illness or accident) or psychological (e.g., birth of a sibling, or parents' divorce). Such beliefs are contrary to research findings and they probably contribute to nurturing feelings of guilt and responsibility that parents have for causing their child's stuttering. In addition, one common belief held in Turkish society is to consider that stuttering is the result of "divine will" (Özdemir, 2010).

During an initial clinical encounter, information on the patient's culture and origins is the object of the clinician's attention to better understand the dynamics in the family with respect to communication (Shapiro, 2011). In highly multilingual countries like Lebanon, it is widely believed that bilingualism causes stuttering. Parents often express the desire to raise their child as monolingual because of this conviction that more than one language may result in confusion for the child, or that it may increase difficulty in word retrieval. Such assumptions regarding bilingualism are often spread broadly on social media or can even be central to advice from some clinicians. Although bingualism is less frequent in Italian and Polish societies, some clinicians not well enough informed regarding causative factors in stuttering may also advise that using one language only is preferable for the dysfluent child.

Early Responses to Beginning Stuttering

Italian, Lebanese, Polish and Turkish parents of children who start to stutter consult initially with their pediatrician, or preschool teacher, who often refer them to clinicians. A matter of concern is that false and misleading information about stuttering (e.g., that it is caused by stress or lack of confidence) is often circulated and perpetuated on the media. Recent studies have shown that both pediatricians (Antoun & Saad Merouwe, 2018) and preschool teachers (Węsierska, et al., 2017) in these countries are not always well-informed about advances in stuttering research and different forms of therapeutic interventions. In fact, preschool teachers may not detect stuttering symptoms easily and are not always knowledgeable about how to deal appropriately with children who stutter, or how to support their parents. They tend to minimise parental concerns and anxiety. Conversely, pediatricians most likely give appropriate general advice to parents and refer them to a clinician, especially if the child stutters severely and the disorder seems to affect the family's quality of life. Some teachers and also some clinicians believe that early stuttering symptoms should be ignored, and that talking about 'the problem' is going to worsen it. In addition, parents may be informed by clinicians that their children are experiencing age-appropriate transient dysfluencies, that are directly linked to language development, and are likely to disappear once language skills improve. In some countries, including Poland, Slovakia, or the Czech Republic, as well as in Lebanon, the term 'physiological stuttering' is sometimes used for this (Lechta, 2010; Tarkowski, et al., 2011). For this reason, many clinicians decide to work on other communication or learning problems instead of implementing stuttering therapy. In the Italian context, children who start stuttering and who tend to withdraw and develop verbal avoidance symptoms are often misdiagnosed. Parents may be advised by clinicians to wait, since stuttering should be allowed to go away on its own. In Turkey and Lebanon specifically, clinical experience shows that fathers are more prone to following the 'wait and see' approach than mothers are. Nevertheless, they often decide to seek the help of a clinician, especially if there is a history of stuttering in the family.

If Italian, Lebanese or Polish clinicians decide to conduct stuttering therapy, in many cases it is limited to counselling parents. However, it is usual for some non-specialist clinicians to start working directly with the child despite the child's lack of stuttering awareness and the absence of a family stuttering history. The direct therapies that are relatively popular in all four countries include fluency shaping methods with strong emphasis on breathing and relaxation techniques. These approaches are often combined with some parental consultation to create a supportive environment for the child. Graduates of the European Clinical Specialization in Fluency are a great support in disseminating knowledge about early stuttering intervention; but, in these countries there is a limited group of these specialists. However, family-based models of stuttering intervention (e.g., the Lidcombe, the Palin PCI, DCM; Guitar & McCauley, 2010) are only being used to a minor degree and primarily by specialised clinicians.

Therapy approaches focusing on reducing environmental triggers, listener reactions, or creating a calmer home environment (e.g., *DCM*, *Palin PCI*) arouse some controversy among parents who often expect that it is the clinician's role 'to fix' their child. In addition, some clinicians do not feel ready to work with parents or even families. For example, Polish clinicians and SLT students report the need for training in counselling, methods to work with the family system and to be able to use some elements of psychotherapeutic approaches in stuttering intervention (Piekacz, et al., 2020). In Italy, there are some integrated approaches that involve working with the child and the parents, and engaging the school, in order to prevent verbal avoidance behaviour (Tomaiuoli, 2009).

Attitudes, Stereotypes and Stigma

Negative attitudes and social stereotypes related to the stutterer, along with the stigma of stuttering, and self-stigma (see Chapter 1), are among the problems that beset people who stutter in all four societies. This means that the person who stutters is at a disadvantage, with unfair judgements regarding negative, undesirable characteristics cast upon them and that stuttering is perceived as 'abnormal' or 'unacceptable' – something that needs to be eliminated. As an example, a 25-year-old Lebanese woman who stutters suggested: *"We are perceived as inferior to other people because we stutter. Therefore, it is very challenging to live in a society like Lebanon where stuttering, or any other difference, is considered as a taboo".* Once associated with a perceived abnormality, the person who stutters experiences awkwardness in expressing or asserting themselves. These feelings lead to negative thoughts and attitudes and the burdensome self-stigma in clients so that they are hampered in developing their potential.

It is not unusual to hear expressions from people who stutter, in all four countries, that include e.g.,: *"I am anxious because I stutter"*, *"I am shy because I stutter"*, *"I am not successful at school because I stutter"* or *"I am not comfortable in social relationships because I stutter"*, *"Everything can be solved if I don't stutter!"* The feeling of being unable to develop potential because they stutter is strong. Also, they feel that they are considered ridiculous, too emotional, unpredictable, or ineffective, and that they want to have better access to certain job positions (Węsierska & Pakura, 2018).

Stereotypical thinking and the social stigma toward stuttering are influential too with regards to choices in therapy alternatives, including group therapy. Parental demand is often for therapy that eliminates atypical dysfluency, because they worry that stuttering will cause limitations to social participation and erect a barrier to realising their children's goals. In patriarchal societies, stuttering in boys is considered devastating because of its influence on their position in society: parents are concerned that stuttering negatively affects suitable employment and marriageability. Similarly, for girls, stuttering is considered a serious flaw.

As a result, non-acceptance of stuttering in society is one of the reasons why some clinicians prefer fluency shaping approaches, use them frequently, even with very young children, and seek zero dysfluencies. One problem with this type of treatment is that its results are hard to maintain, and relapses have dire consequences on the individual's self-efficacy.

Some clinicians maintain that stuttering must be eliminated at any cost since listening to someone's stuttering can be burdensome for fluent speakers. Misinformation and stigma drive many clients to consult with professionals with limited expertise in the field, or those who promise 'a quick cure' for stuttering after a reduced number of therapy sessions or intensive residential therapy programs. Since SLT as a profession is relatively new in these countries, there are still other professionals (special education teachers, medical doctors, psychologists, psychotherapists) providing stuttering therapy. They mainly aim for fluent speech and a complete cure of stuttering within a couple of weeks. Although the number of specialised clinicians is increasing rapidly in these countries, the claims of the non-specialised professionals and their unrealistic promises affect the overall therapy expectations of the families of children and adults who stutter. It is also apparent that speech-language therapists are still perceived as the professionals who should deal with the technical, speech motor related aspects of communication; whereas psychologists are usually expected to take over the affective and cognitive areas of stuttering.

Preference for Fluency Shaping Approaches

By consulting clinicians, Lebanese and Polish clients and/or their families commonly ask for a total "cure" for stuttering. As non-acceptance of stuttering contributes to the preference for fluency shaping approaches.

Many clinicians in the four countries are learning contemporary methods of stuttering intervention either by means of formal academic education or through additional training courses. It is common that clinicians try to combine different therapy approaches by using stuttering modification and speech restructuring approaches to respond to the client's needs. However, many do not feel confident enough to work on cognition and emotions, so they are likely to refer the client to a psychologist to work simultaneously on these components. Often, the only support available for Polish adults is to join informal self-help groups for people who stutter (Węsierska & Pakura, 2018).

Self-help Groups

In general, clinicians acknowledge that self-help groups for people who stutter support them on many different levels. Sharing stories of experiences, managing the negative attitudes of some listeners and looking to begin changing attitudes, including self-stigma, are among the advantages of self-help groups (see Chapter 1). The Polish self-help stuttering movement has a relatively long history and is well established (Jankowska-Szafarska, 2017; Węsierska, & Pakura, 2018). There is a nationwide association (*Ostoja*) (http://jakanielublin.pl/) and there are also several non-profit organisations that support them. In almost every main Polish city there are self-help groups called *Kluby J.*, that cater for adults. The situation is slightly less favorable regarding children and their parents, but support groups are just beginning to emerge. In Turkey, the self-help group movement is growing, in parallel to the speech-language pathology area. Although a decade ago a group of clinicians tried to organise a web-based self-help initiative in Turkey (St. Louis, Topbas, & Özdemir 2008), the official self-help organisation was not established until 2017. The Association of People Who Stutter (*Kekemeler Derneği*) aims "to create social awareness about stuttering and to protect the economic, social and cultural interests of people who stutter" (http://kekemelerdernegi.com). They have organised self-help group meetings in around 40 cities and sometimes clinicians take part in them. As in Poland, mostly adults attend these gatherings but, in some instances, children and their families participate. Moreover, the Polish and Turkish associations have organised conferences and initiated campaigns to increase public awareness and provide information about stuttering.

Unlike Poland and Turkey, self-help groups are not yet flourishing in Italy and Lebanon. In Italy, people who stutter do meet to support each other, but often as venues for finding solutions to stop stuttering. Attempts by some Lebanese clinicians to bring adult clients together to encourage establishment of a self-help group have been unsuccessful, and the group ceased to exist once the clinicians withdrew. A potential explanation is the level of negative stereotyping of stuttering in Lebanon, as clients show reluctance even to attend group therapy in clinical settings.

Therapeutic Intervention Suggestions

Given the commonalities among the four cultures regarding how stuttering and therapy are viewed, clinicians have starting points for discussion with parents and clients, and can be prepared to be open and informative about stuttering and about what therapy can and cannot offer. Discussion regarding parental and client priorities, along with management of the therapy process are important, as well as clinicians being mindful about their own cultural stereotyping (e.g., clinician assumptions about gender or role assignments in some societies). While working with clients coming from Lebanon and Turkey specifically, it is good to take enough time to discuss the beliefs that adults who stutter or the parents of children who stutter have about the aetiology of stuttering and to provide scientifically proven answers to all their questions. Clinical experience reveals that the better informed the clients and/ or parents are, the more they trust the clinician and engage in therapy. Listening to client concerns and showing them understanding are key elements for therapeutic alliance. With preschoolers, working with parents is not always an easy task because they often expect that it is the clinician who must 'fix' the stuttering. Therefore, clinicians need to explain the reasons for engaging parents in therapy, and to refer to scientific evidence in support of their clinical decisions.

Parental roles and family involvement in therapy are areas that require clinicians to be sensitive yet open in discussion regarding how best to organise working with the child who stutters. In Lebanon and in Turkey for instance, when both parents are invited to attend, it is important to engage them both from the beginning: via eye contact and addressing questions directly to fathers as well as to mothers. Quite often to create a supportive environment, clinicians work with the entire family, which comprises the extended family members, so their involvement is important too. Some family members will have specific concerns or advice that needs to be discussed, so that the family can agree on therapeutic decisions to help the child that guides them towards different therapeutic goals: for example, teaching fluency techniques to young children may be a concern of some family members that can be considered in light of alternatives that direct attention to the child's increasing confidence in communicating.

To reduce the reluctance or apprehension that some adults have regarding joining group therapy, gradual preparation through reading or watching videos of group therapy involvement and looking at the advantages of this kind of experience is likely to be more effective for Lebanese adults. Meeting one or two others who stutter for coffee can open the door to discussing self-help group meetings.

In Italy, becoming more effective communicators regardless of dysfluencies has to be increasingly emphasised to become the main goal of therapy. No less important is to devote as many resources as possible to inform the client about the origin of stuttering and to fully share the realistic goals of effective therapy. Collaboration and a meaningful environment, including available group support, are crucial for the purpose of gaining acceptance and trust in the therapeutic process. Very often parents come to the clinician hoping to have a confirmation of what the pediatrician's recommendation is, for example: "there is no need to intervene, and you have to relax". When a child is stuttering, such reasoning can be ineffective and can seem to relieve parents from responsibility to be engaged with therapy, rather than delegating the responsibility completely to the clinician and not be involved.

Working with Polish people who stutter and their families can raise particular issues that need consideration. One is that parents typically blame themselves for their child's stuttering. Parents of young children are very frequently confused due to conflicting information about the causes of stuttering or how best to support their child's communication. When risk factors for stuttering in a child accumulate and the clinician is discussing the chances of persistence of stuttering, this is typically difficult for parents to accept since they expect stuttering to be eradicated. Concerning school-age children, it is imperative to convince parents to participate in the therapy process and cooperate with the school environment.

In the case of adolescents, the problem may be their resistance to starting therapy and parental pressure. Parents are not always open to discuss with their older children regarding what should happen in the therapy process. Polish parents tend to adopt authoritative and/or overprotective attitudes towards their adolescents; this is similar to attitudes of Italian parents. In such situations, it can be helpful to share information on the psychological determinants of adolescent behaviour (Ficek, Jeziorczak & Węsierska, 2021). It can be beneficial to present the stages of the transtheoretical change model in stuttering therapy (see also chapter 2; and Floyd, et al., 2007). Using this model can increase parents' understanding of the importance of their child's willingness to undertake therapy and take responsibility for its progress.

Additionally, the unrealistic expectations of the therapy process coming from adults who stutter may be a challenge for clinicians. Helping clients to express their feelings and thoughts about communication and stuttering and to verbalise their ideas and expectations may significantly increase the effectiveness of therapeutic intervention. It may happen that they insist on trying certain techniques and if they are not completely satisfied, they are usually ready to attempt something new. Therefore, sharing the knowledge, and desensitising them toward stuttering can become essential parts to the therapy process.

Conclusion

This chapter explores multicultural considerations that are important in stuttering intervention in Italy, Lebanon, Poland and Turkey. Multicultural awareness drives clinicians to value human diversity in all its forms and to approach clients and their families as individuals with similarities and differences. Hence, it is fundamental to disseminate reliable knowledge about stuttering and how to effectively support people who experience limitations in everyday communication. Further, informing potential therapy recipients about the realistic therapy goals and the relevant evidence-based methods will serve to achieve them. The World Health Organization's International Classification of Functioning, Disability, and Health – ICF (World Health Organization, 2001; Yaruss & Quesal, 2004) is an excellent tool for the diagnosis and for therapeutic process in order to remove barriers to activities and participation. This ICF model is gradually becoming recognised and recommended in these countries (Faściszewska, 2019; Saad-Merouwe, 2020, Tomaiuoli, 2021).

It is clear that the four cultures discussed in this chapter share many commonalities (including certain uninformed beliefs about stuttering, negative attitudes and social stigma, and preference for particular approaches); however, they differ in the advancement of self-help groups (established and flourishing in Poland and Turkey, in contrast to Italy and Lebanon).

In conclusion, for the four countries, building a good relationship with clients and parents based on mutual respect, knowledge and information sharing are crucial from the beginning of the therapy process. The more knowledgeable that clients and parents are, the more open to collaboration they will be. It is equally vital for clinicians to listen empathetically to clients and parents without judging them. Clinicians can expect better outcomes in the therapeutic process if they can demonstrate their ability to support their clients and their families to become aware of their resources and potentials.

In summary, one of the most difficult challenges in the four countries is to develop the clients' willingness to confront and to accept their stuttering. When the stereotype regarding stuttering is strong within a community, many who stutter will also have their self-stigma to manage, so such acceptance is difficult. Applying the small steps rule, and where possible engaging in group support are extremely beneficial to the success of the therapeutic intervention. As in many other societies, providing appropriate local education and spreading information in the clients' environment and among members of society generally are essential to reduce the stigma and negative stereotyping related to people who stutter.

References

Antoun, G. & Saad Merouwe, S. (2018). *Le bégaiement dans la petite enfance: état des lieux des connaissances des pédiatres au Liban*. Unpublished Bachelor degree thesis, Beirut: Université Saint-Joseph.

Bloodstein, O., Bernstein Ratner, N., & Brundage S. B. (2021). *The handbook on stuttering* (7th Ed.). San Diego, CA: Plural Publishing Inc.

Błachnio, A., Przepiórka A., St. Louis K. O., Węsierska M., & Węsierska K. (2015). Postawy społeczne wobec jąkania w Polsce – przegląd. In K. Węsierska (Ed.), *Zaburzenia płynności mowy: teoria i praktyka. Tom 1* (pp. 89–100). Katowice: Komlogo – Uniwersytet Śląski.

Faściszewska, M. (2019). Diagnoza utrwalonego jąkania z wykorzystaniem klasyfikacji ICF. *Forum Logopedy*. 31, 4–9.

Ficek, E., Jeziorczak, B., & Węsierska, K. (2021). Poradnictwo logopedyczne dla osób jąkających się i ich rodzin. In K. Węsierska, & H. Sønsterud, (Eds.), *Dialog bez barier – kompleksowa interwencja logopedyczna w jąkaniu. Wydanie polskie rozszerzone* (pp. 85–115). Chorzów: Agere Aude.

Floyd, J., Zebrowski, P. M., & Flamme, G. A. (2007). Stages of change and stuttering: A preliminary view. *Journal of Fluency Disorders*. 23, 1–30. 10.1016/j.jfludis.2007.03.001

Guitar, B. & McCauley, R. (2010). *Treatment of stuttering. Established and Emerging Interventions*. Baltimore: Lippincott Williams & Wilkins.

Jankowska-Szafarska, L. (2017). Co działa w samopomocy? Szeroka perspektywa. In. L. Jankowska-Szafarska, B. Suligowska, R., Kara, K. Kupiec (Eds.), *Życie z zacięciem. Integralny przewodnik po jąkaniu* (pp. 269–275). Kraków: Wydawnictwo Edukacyjne.

Kakareko, A. (2017). Moje życie z "j". In. L. Jankowska-Szafarska, B. Suligowska, R., Kara, & K. Kupiec (Eds.), *Życie z zacięciem. Integralny przewodnik po jąkaniu* (pp. 223–227). Kraków: Wydawnictwo Edukacyjne.

Lechta, V. (2010). *Koktavost. Integrativní přístup*. Praha: Portál.

Özdemir, R. S. (2010). *Measuring public attitudes toward stuttering: Eskişehir sample*. Unpublished PhD thesis, Eskişehir: Anadolu University.

Piekacz, P., Węsierska, K., & Wesierska, M. (2020). Uwarunkowania skuteczności utrwalonego jąkania w opiniach logopedów i studentów logopedii. *Logopaedica Lodziensia*. 4, 187–204.

Polish Association of People Who Stutter "Ostoja": http://jakanielublin.pl/ (Accessed: 29 October 2021).

Shapiro, D. (2011). *Stuttering intervention: A collaborative journey to fluency freedom* (2nd Ed.), Texas: Pro-Ed.

Saad-Merouwe, S. (2020). Terapia dopasowana do potrzeb osoby jąkającej się – studium przypadku. In K. Węsierska & M. Witkowski (Eds.), *Zaburzenia płynności mowy: teoria i praktyka. Tom 2* (pp. 205–222). Katowice: Uniwersytet Śląski.

St. Louis, K. O., Topbas, S., & Özdemir, R. S. (2008). Turkish Stuttering Association: A model project to bring stuttering self-help to Turkey. *Perspectives on Fluency and Fluency Disorders*. 18 (3), 119–123. 10.1044/ffd18.3.119

Tarkowski, Z., Humeniuk, E., & Dunaj, J. (2011). *Jąkanie w wieku przedszkolnym*. Olsztyn: Wydawnictwo UWM.

The Association of People Who Stutter (Turkey): http://kekemelerdernegi.com (Accessed: 12 April 2021).

Tomaiuoli D. (2009). *Favolando con la balbuzie dei piccolo*. Roma: SEU.

Tomaiuoli D. (2021). *Balbuzie in adolescenza*. Trento: Edizioni Erickson.

Turnbull, A. P., Turnbull, R., Erwin, E. J., & Soodak, L. C. (2006). *Families, professionals, and exceptionality: Positive outcomes through partnerships and trust* (5th Ed.). Upper Saddle River, NJ: Prentice Hall.

Węsierska, K., Laszczyńska, A., & Pakura, M. (2017). Wczesna interwencja w jąkaniu wczesnodziecięcym w Polsce – w opiniach logopedów i rodziców dzieci jąkających się. *Forum Logopedyczne*. 25, 81–96.

Węsierska, K. & Pakura, M. (2018). Sytuacja dorosłych zmagających się z jąkaniem w Polsce w opiniach logopedów i osób jąkających się. In K. Węsierska & K. Gaweł (Eds.), *Zaburzenia płynności mowy* (pp. 113–130). Gdańsk: Wydawnictwo Harmonia Universalis.

World Health Organization (2001). International classification of functioning, disability and health: ICF. World Health Organization. https://apps.who.int/iris/handle/10665/42407

Yaruss, J. S., & Quesal, R. W. (2004). Stuttering and the international classification of functioning, disability, and health (ICF): An update. *Journal of Communication Disorders*. 37, 35–52.

12 Acquired Stuttering

Catherine Theys and John A. Tetnowski

Introduction

Stuttering is a speech fluency disorder characterised by the occurrence of *stuttering dysfluencies*. These dysfluencies are the core behaviours of stuttering and include part-word repetitions, single syllable word repetitions, prolongations and blocks. Stuttering can also be associated with secondary behaviours and negative affective and cognitive thoughts. In the literature, the term stuttering is often used as a synonym for developmental stuttering. However, not all stuttering is developmental in origin.

Stuttering can also have an onset following cerebrovascular injuries, traumatic brain injuries, neurodegenerative conditions and emotional traumas. This has been described in the literature as late-onset stuttering or adult-onset stuttering, among other terms (De Nil et al., 2017). For the purpose of this chapter, we will use the wording *acquired stuttering* to differentiate it from *developmental stuttering*. This terminology is preferred as acquired stuttering can also have an onset in childhood due to a neurological or psychological trauma, although such conditions are more likely to appear later in life (Theys & De Nil, in press).

The International Classification of Disease has categorised the different types of stuttering (World Health Organization, 2018; see Table 12.1). In this chapter, we will refer to childhood onset fluency disorder (F80.81) as *developmental stuttering*, to stuttering following neurological events (I69) or disorders (R47.82) as *acquired neurogenic stuttering* and to stuttering following emotional trauma (F98.5) as *acquired functional stuttering*. The term functional has gradually replaced the term psychogenic, as it allows focusing on the behavioural symptoms that are present, rather than on the presumed underlying aetiology of the speech problem (Edwards et al., 2014). Further, it should be noted that stuttering can also be *malingered*, as opposed to *acquired*. Malingering is the feigning of a condition, typically for financial or some other type of gain (Bass & Halligan, 2014) and is classified in the ICF as Z76.5.

DOI: 10.4324/9781003179016-12

Table 12.1 International Classification of Disease classifications for stuttering

Code	Description	Inclusion
F80.81	childhood onset fluency disorder	• stuttering; cluttering • childhood onset
F98.5	adult onset fluency disorder	• stuttering • adult onset • other emotional/psychogenic
I69	fluency disorder (stuttering) following cerebrovascular disease	• stuttering, dysfluency • stroke, traumatic brain injury, vascular/circulatory disease
R47.82	fluency disorder in conditions classified elsewhere	• stuttering, dysfluency • Parkinson's, Tourette's

Current State of the Art

Acquired stuttering can be neurogenic or functional in origin. Our knowledge of these acquired types of stuttering has significantly increased – and changed – over the past 20 years. We will provide a brief overview of the current state of knowledge here, but readers are referred elsewhere for more detailed recent overviews (De Nil et al., 2017; Duffy, 2020; Theys & De Nil, in press).

Approximately half of the cases of acquired neurogenic stuttering are caused by stroke. This is followed by traumatic brain injuries and neurodegenerative diseases such as Parkinson's and Alzheimer's disease (Lundgren et al., 2010; Theys et al., 2008). The onset of acquired neurogenic stuttering has also been linked with many other conditions that may influence brain functioning, including deep brain stimulation and use of medication (Brady, 1998; Picillo et al., 2017). Most people with acquired neurogenic stuttering will not have a history of developmental stuttering, but it is possible that pre-existing stuttering may re-occur following neurological conditions (Helm-Estabrooks, 1999). Detailed prevalence data is sparse, but one study showed that 5% of 319 stroke patients presented with >3% stuttering dysfluencies in the acute phase following stroke. While some recovered from their stuttering, follow-up after 6 months showed that stuttering persisted in eight of 14 patients who were re-assessed (Theys et al., 2011). Studies on Parkinson's disease suggest that the prevalence ranges from 4–57% (Hartelius, 2015; Whitfield et al., 2018), with the large variability possibly due to differences in disease progression and differences in diagnostic criteria used.

Acquired functional stuttering can occur as a psychological reaction to stress or trauma. It often occurs without evidence of an underlying neurological disease, although 20 of 69 patients with functional stuttering in Baumgartner and Duffy's (1997) study had evidence of neurological disease. While precise prevalence data is again not available, stuttering occurred in 53% of 30 patients with functional speech and voice disorders (Baizabal-Carvallo & Jankovic, 2015).

Contrary to previous beliefs, these prevalence numbers indicate that acquired stuttering is not rare. However, clients with acquired stuttering may not always receive referrals for speech therapy support for their fluency problems.

Traditionally, a number of features were suggested to differentiate acquired neurogenic stuttering from functional and developmental stuttering in adults (i.e., consistency of stuttering across speech tasks, dysfluencies not restricted to content words or word-initial positions and absence of anxiety, secondary symptoms and adaptation effect, Helm-Estabrooks, 1999). However, use of these criteria may lead to underdiagnosis as these features do not apply to all – or some even to most – clients with acquired neurogenic stuttering (Market et al., 1990; Stewart & Rowley, 1996; Theys et al., 2008). Recent evidence shows that stuttering characteristics vary depending on the underlying aetiology of acquired neurogenic stuttering, and it is therefore important not to overgeneralise findings across aetiologies. For example, dysfluencies in neurogenic stuttering following stroke occur almost always in initial position (De Nil et al., 2017) and the location of within-utterance dysfluencies does not differ from developmental stuttering (Max et al., 2019). Reading adaptation occurs in about half of the clients with stuttering following stroke and TBI (De Nil et al., 2017; Jokel et al., 2007) and in at least two thirds of people with stuttering following Parkinson's disease (Whitfield et al., 2018). Most reports across all acquired neurogenic stuttering aetiologies indicate increased fluency when singing. Approximately half of the cases in the literature on neurogenic stuttering following stroke report presence of secondary behaviours (e.g., facial grimacing, fist clenching), and more than two thirds show negative speech-associated emotions (Theys & De Nil, in press). A similarly high occurrence of secondary behaviours and emotions has been reported following traumatic brain injury, but these behaviours seem to occur less frequently in clients with an onset of stuttering following neurodegenerative conditions (Theys et al., 2008).

Acquired functional stuttering may present with characteristics similar to those seen in developmental and acquired neurogenic stuttering. However, the speech characteristics are often described as atypical. Atypical may refer to the pattern of dysfluencies (e.g., very consistent on each syllable), the location of the dysfluencies (e.g., word-initial as well as word-final), the variation in dysfluencies (e.g., change in dysfluency types throughout a conversation) and suggestibility (e.g., change in stuttering severity consistent with clinician suggestion of task difficulty). People with acquired functional stuttering seem to adapt less, with one in nine clients showing reading adaptation in Baumgartner and Duffy's (1997) study. The most striking feature of acquired functional stuttering is the ability to achieve a very rapid (1–2 sessions) improvement in fluency (in 70% of cases) (Baumgartner & Duffy, 1997). However, as with acquired neurogenic stuttering, the stuttering characteristics can vary widely across individuals.

Differential Diagnosis

The information presented earlier shows that – besides the core stuttering dysfluencies – there are no defining characteristics that apply to each person with acquired stuttering. The diagnostic process will therefore need to be tailored to each individual client, taking underlying conditions and co-occurring speech, language and cognitive problems into account. If the stuttering occurs later in life, in a person who previously spoke fluently, the acquired as opposed to developmental onset of stuttering is usually clear. More important is the differentiation between neurogenic and functional aetiologies of acquired stuttering as these will have direct implications for treatment. Another important differentiation to make is that between acquired neurogenic stuttering following events such as stroke and traumatic brain injury, where an improvement in symptoms can be expected, and stuttering associated with neurodegenerative conditions, where a progressive worsening of the stuttering needs to be anticipated.

Many clients with acquired stuttering will present with a complex combination of symptoms. In addition to a comprehensive fluency assessment, assessment for other communication and cognitive difficulties may be necessary. All stuttering/fluency assessments should begin with collection of accurate case history information, an assessment and description of speech characteristics across tasks of varying length, complexity and settings and an assessment of attitudes about stuttering. This needs to be followed by trialling of potential therapeutic interventions, such as fluency-inducing tasks (e.g., prolonged speech, singing, pacing, reading adaptation, delayed auditory feedback). This type of complete evaluation can help in both differential diagnosis and planning of intervention. An example of a comprehensive fluency profile is provided in the online resources.

Treatment Options

If the assessment results uncover that stuttering is perceived as a significant problem by the client, specific treatment for the stuttering needs to be provided. This does not always happen, as the two cases described in the following sections were initially not referred for stuttering therapy, despite stuttering being their most prominent and disabling communication problem.

Before starting stuttering therapy, it is important to note that some clients with acquired stuttering following stroke may recover spontaneously, and sometimes more pressing medical issues need to be prioritised. Due to the often-complex presentation of problems, a multidisciplinary approach may be needed. In some cases, adjusting medication (Brady, 1998) or deep brain stimulation parameters (Picillo et al., 2017) may be sufficient to alleviate the stuttering. Other important considerations include quality of life and inclusion of family members in decision-making.

There are no evidence-based speech treatments that have been developed specifically for acquired neurogenic stuttering. However, our clinical experiences indicate that an individualised approach is necessary and a variety of speech therapy approaches have been reported to be successful. These include fluency shaping, stuttering modification, rhythmic speech or slowing down the speech rate. Success with altered auditory feedback and pacing strategies has also been described (Theys & De Nil, in press).

For people with acquired functional stuttering, discussing the absence of a neurological problem that may hinder progress is often helpful, as is directly addressing the underlying psychological problem (e.g., with psychological counselling or using cognitive strategies) and using fluency-inducing techniques to help clients 'find' their fluent speech again. In clinical settings, this is accomplished through accurate assessment of all information gathered and reported, followed by a frank and honest debriefing with the client and their family. As described earlier, rapid recovery occurs often, and clients may need support in explaining such a rapid change to family and others in their environment (Duffy, 2020).

Many of these considerations are reflected in the two cases presented here.

Case # 1

MB was presented to one of the authors (JT) at a university speech and hearing clinic. MB initially came to the clinic with reported symptoms of aphasia. She was subsequently referred for a fluency evaluation during the course of her initial visit.

MB was in her early 50's when she had a sudden onset of stuttering. The stuttering started two months before the initial evaluation, after a spell of dizziness and weakness, with brief loss of consciousness. When she awoke, she could not speak at first. When she finally could speak, she presented with severe stuttering. There was no stuttering in her history prior to this point in time and an MRI revealed no new damage. She previously had a diagnosis of breast cancer at age 40 and had two subsequent bouts with cancer. Four months prior to her stuttering onset, she received chemotherapy and carried a post-therapy diagnosis of chemo-induced neuropathy.

MB's fluency evaluation (using the format in Appendix 12.A) revealed several key findings. These included: 10% stuttered syllables during word tasks and 13% during conversation. Stuttering types included part-word repetitions and blocks that ranged between 1–3 seconds in duration. Stuttering dysfluencies occurred on content and function words and in phrase initial and phrase medial points. No secondary behaviours were noted. Fluency-inducing tasks including prolonged speech, mouthed speech, whispering and singing resulted in no change in stuttering. She was administered the Overall Assessment of the Speaker's Experience of Stuttering (Yaruss & Quesal, 2006) and showed a mild, but significant reaction to her stuttering. One item of note was her substituting of words when she feared stuttering. During the evaluation (and during subsequent early therapy sessions) she often cried when she stuttered. In addition, she showed mild word finding difficulties. She scored in the low, but normal range of the Boston Naming Test (Goodglass et al., 1983). A sample of her speech at this time is provided in Audio 12.1.

MB was enrolled in therapy. Fluency enhancing techniques (prolonged speech, increased pauses) were the dominant philosophy during the initial three months of therapy with little success and significant frustration. This appears in Audio 12.2. After a thorough case review, it was decided that there was a significant emotional component attached to her stuttering, and her therapy was modified to more of a stuttering modification approach where her therapy emphasised education about stuttering, decreasing word substitutions and building communication confidence. At this point in time, she was made aware that her diagnosis of stuttering was modified from *neurogenic* to "*psychogenic*". Although initially upset, MB was counselled to understand that she could indeed control her speech and that it was not due to neurogenic limitations. She embraced this view with counselling from the clinician and was dismissed from therapy two months after the shift in diagnosis and treatment paradigm. At the time of dismissal, MB demonstrated less than 1% stuttering dysfluencies at word tasks and 2% during conversation tasks (Audio 12.3). Her OASES score was very mild.

In summary, this case shows how – despite the diagnosis of chemotherapy-induced neuropathy – MB fit the updated criteria for acquired functional stuttering. Proper differential diagnosis allowed for more of a counselling and acceptance method of intervention with a successful outcome within a few months.

Case # 2

Similar to Case #1, DB was referred to a university speech and hearing clinic to participate in aphasia groups. However, she decided not to attend these groups due to embarrassment about her speech problems and was referred to one of the authors (CT) for a fluency assessment.

DB was 79-years-old when she had a left occipital infarct. This was followed by an additional left total anterior circulation stroke one month later and multiple post-stroke epileptic seizures. She spoke fluently before these events, as can be seen in Video 12.1. Following the strokes and seizures, DB was diagnosed with receptive and expressive aphasia, apraxia of speech, speech dysfluencies and cognitive problems. Our initial stuttering assessment took place 5 months following onset of the seizures.

During two baseline assessment sessions, DB presented with 41% and 39% stuttered syllables during spontaneous speech, respectively. Her stuttering dysfluencies consisted of repetitions of sounds, syllables, monosyllabic words and blocks. An example of her pre-treatment speech can be seen in Video 12.2. During the assessment sessions, a number of different treatment techniques were trialled. Her speech fluency increased markedly during singing, unison speech and repetition. This is illustrated in Video 12.3. DB also presented with secondary behaviours, such as clenching her jaw and fists during stuttering dysfluencies. She reacted verbally to her dysfluencies and reported to be frustrated and embarrassed about 'getting stuck', which had led to social isolation.

One-hour treatment sessions were started, once per week. She completed two 10-week treatment blocks, with a 5-month break in between due to personal events in the client's life. During the assessment sessions, it became evident that the combination of speech, language and cognitive problems required a stuttering treatment approach that that would require minimal cognitive demands. The paced speech approach was most successful, especially when supported with visual and tactile feedback given by a pacing board, and visual and auditory guidance given by the clinician. The client was encouraged to tap a square on a laminated six-square pacing board, with her index finger, for each syllable she produced. As she spontaneously started tapping a square for each word rather than syllable, we adjusted our approach to what came most natural to her. During the training phase, frequent modelling of pacing board use was provided. The clinician demonstrated using the pacing board and then tapped along with the participant. When the participant was able to use the technique independently without clinician modelling, external guiding from the clinician was gradually removed.

Once the pacing technique was implemented successfully, it was complemented with low-level cognitive restructuring to address the negative emotions and attitudes around communication. Strategies were implemented to recognise and reduce frustration. These included pausing, self-imposed time out, relaxation through deep breathing and easy onset. Next, naming tasks were introduced as word finding problems were the second most frequent cause for interruptions in speech fluency following the stuttering dysfluencies. We focused on names and relationships of DB's family members as talking with and about her family were priorities for her. At the start of the second treatment block, a goal of increased participation in community activities was set following a shared goal-setting approach. Treatment focused on skill transfer and generalisation, and conversation partner training was implemented. This included instructed demonstration of the techniques to ensure that the conversation partners would continue to provide support and reminders outside of the therapy sessions, when needed.

During the first treatment block, DB's stuttering frequency during spontaneous speech decreased from 41% to 24% stuttered syllables. An example of DB using the pacing technique at the end of this treatment block can be seen in Video 12.4. During the treatment break, DB reported not to have worked on her speech as she had been faced with significant personal loss. Her stuttering frequency had increased to 66% at the start of the second treatment block. However, it quickly reduced following re-introduction of the techniques and returned to 22% during the final session.

As DB's stuttering frequency decreased throughout both treatment blocks, her reactions to the stuttering also decreased. As the second treatment block progressed, DB began attending social activities in the retirement village as well as weekly gym classes. She also commented on improvement in her confidence and increased willingness to engage with others. Overall, the treatment resulted in a significant improvement in DB's quality of life.

Summary and Clinical Implications

Acquired stuttering is characterised by the occurrence of stuttering dys-fluencies in a person's speech, and these can be secondary to acquired neurogenic conditions or can be functional in origin. The stuttering dys-fluencies are the core characteristic of acquired stuttering, and presence of other characteristics (e.g., emotional reactions) can vary depending on the underlying aetiology and client characteristics. Differential diagnosis be-tween neurogenic and functional stuttering needs to be attempted – al-though this may need to be adjusted later on as more information becomes available. A detailed assessment session is also needed to provide informa-tion regarding potential treatment strategies.

The two cases presented here both had a complex medical history and were initially not referred for stuttering therapy, despite the stuttering being their most significant communication problem. For both clients, different treatment approaches were trialled and gradually adjusted over the course of the treat-ment. While both had a different underlying aetiology of their acquired stuttering (neurogenic versus functional), they showed a large and clinically meaningful reduction in stuttering dysfluencies and a significant improvement in quality of life following treatment.

These cases illustrate the importance of recognising acquired stuttering dysfluencies as a problem that may require specific stuttering treatment, and such treatment should be provided upon the client's request. Despite the shortage of evidence-based therapy information in the literature, the cases presented here show that individualised treatment approaches can lead to positive outcomes.

References

Baizabal-Carvallo, J. & Jankovic, J. (2015) Speech and voice disorders in patients with psy-chogenic movement disorders. *Journal of Neurology*. 262, 2420–2424. 10.1007/s00415-015-7856-7

Bass, C. D. & Halligan, P. P. (2014) Factitious disorders and malingering: challenges for clinical assessment and management. *The Lancet (British Edition)*. 383(9926), 1422–1432. 10.1016/S0140-6736(13)62186-8

Baumgartner, J. & Duffy, J. R. (1997) Psychogenic stuttering in adults with and without neurologic disease. *Journal of Medical Speech Language Pathology*. 5, 75–96.

Brady, J. P. (1998) Drug-induced stuttering: A review of the literature. *Journal of Clinical Psychopharmacology.* 18(1), 50–54. 10.1097/00004714-199802000-00008

De Nil, L. F., Theys, C. & Jokel, R. (2017) Stroke-related acquired neurogenic stuttering. In: Coppens, P., (ed.), *Aphasia Rehabilitation: Clinical Challenges.* Burlington, MA: Jones & Bartlett Learning, 173–202.

Duffy, J. R. (2020) *Motor speech disorders: substrates, differential diagnosis, and management.* 4th ed. St. Louis, Missouri: Elsevier.

Edwards, M. J., Stone, J. & Lang, A. E. (2014) From psychogenic movement disorder to functional movement disorder: it's time to change the name. *Movement Disorders.* 29(7), 849–852. 10.1002/mds.25562

Goodglass, H., Kaplan, E. & Weintraub, S. (1983) *Boston Naming Test.* Philadelphia, PA: Lea & Febiger.

Hartelius, L. (2015) Incidence of Developmental Speech Dysfluencies in Individuals with Parkinson's Disease. *Folia Phoniatrica et Logopaedica.* 66(3), 132–137. 10.1159/000368751

Helm-Estabrooks, N. (1999) Stuttering associated with acquired neurological disorders. *Stuttering and Related Disorders of Fluency.* 3, 255–268.

Jokel, R., De Nil, L. & Sharpe, K. (2007) Speech disfluencies in adults with neurogenic stuttering associated with stroke and traumatic brain injury. *Journal of Medical Speech-Language Pathology.* 15(3), 243–262.

Lundgren, K., Helm-Estabrooks, N. & Klein, R. (2010) Stuttering following acquired brain damage: A review of the literature. *Journal of Neurolinguistics.* 23(5), 447–454. 10.1016/j.jneuroling.2009.08.008

Market, K. E., Montague, J. C., Buffalo, M. D. & Drummond, S. S. (1990) Acquired stuttering: Descriptive data and treatment outcome. *Journal of Fluency Disorders.* 15(1), 21–33. 10.1016/0094-730X(90)90029-R

Max, L., Kadri, M., Mitsuya, T. & Balasubramanian, V. (2019) Similar within-utterance loci of dysfluency in acquired neurogenic and persistent developmental stuttering. *Brain and Language.* 189, 1–9. 10.1016/0094-730X(90)90029-R

Picillo, M., Vincos, G. B., Sammartino, F., Lozano, A. M. & Fasano, A. (2017) Exploring risk factors for stuttering development in Parkinson disease after deep brain stimulation. *Parkinsonism & Related Disorders.* 38, 85–89. 10.1016/j.parkreldis.2017.02.015

Stewart, T. & Rowley, D. (1996) Acquired stammering in Great Britain. *International Journal of Language & Communication Disorders.* 31(1), 1–9. 10.3109/13682829609033148

Swinburn, K., Porter, G. & Howard, D. (2005) *Comprehensive Aphasia Test,* Taylor & Francis.

Theys, C. & De Nil, L. F. (in press) Acquired stuttering: etiology, symptomatology, identification and treatment. In Zebrowski, P., Anderson, J. & Conture, E., (eds.), *Stuttering: Characteristics, Assessment and Treatment.* 4th ed. Thieme Publishers.

Theys, C., Van Wieringen, A. & De Nil, L. F. (2008) A clinician survey of speech and non-speech characteristics of neurogenic stuttering. *Journal of Fluency Disorders.* 33(1), 1–23. 10.1016/j.jfludis.2007.09.001

Theys, C., van Wieringen, A., Sunaert, S., Thijs, V. & De Nil, L. F. (2011) A one year prospective study of neurogenic stuttering following stroke: Incidence and co-occurring disorders. *Journal of Communication Disorders.* 44(6), 678–687. 10.1016/j.jcomdis.2011.06.001

Whitfield, J. A., Delong, C., Goberman, A. M. & Blomgren, M. (2018) Fluency adaptation in speakers with Parkinson disease: a motor learning perspective. *International Journal of Speech Language Pathology*, 20(7), 699–707. 10.1080/17549507.2017.1341549

World Health Organization (2018) *International Classification of Diseases for Mortality and Morbidity Statistics (11th Revision).*

Yaruss, J. S. & Quesal, R. W. (2006) Overall Assessment of the Speaker's Experience of Stuttering (OASES): Documenting multiple outcomes in stuttering treatment. *Journal of Fluency Disorders.* 31(2), 90–115. 10.1016/j.jfludis.2006.02.002

Index

For Product Safety Concerns and Information please contact our EU
representative GPSR@taylorandfrancis.com
Taylor & Francis Verlag GmbH, Kaufingerstraße 24, 80331 München, Germany